Pearls from a Pediatric Practice

Frank Oski (Contemporary Pediatrics)

James A. Stockman (Yearbook of Pediatrics)

Thomas Frist, Sr.   Pete Riley   My Wife (Anna)

Audio Digest Tapes   CDC Reports

My Four Grandchildren (Mallie, Kelly, Colson, Mazi)

St. Louis Children's Hospital   My Patients

My Four Children
(Amy, Van,
John, Jeff)

Sydney Gellis (Pediatric Notes)

James Overall   Barton Schmitt

Medical Students   Richard Goodbloom

Pediatric Annals   Colleagues   Amos Christie

Vanderbilt Children's Hospital

Pearls *from a* Pediatric Practice I

William Wadlington, MD
Clinical Professor of Pediatrics
Vanderbilt University
School of Medicine
Nashville, Tennessee

and

Clifton K. Meador, MD
Chief Medical Officer
Saint Thomas Hospital
Clinical Professor of Medicine
Vanderbilt University
School of Medicine
Nashville, Tennessee

HANLEY & BELFUS, INC.
Philadelphia

Published by HANLEY & BELFUS, INC., Medical Publishers,
210 South 13th Street, Philadelphia, PA 19107.
215-546-7293; 800-962-1892; fax 215-790-9330.
Website: www.hanleyandbelfus.com

For information about ordering bulk quantities of the book for educational purposes, contact the publisher at 215-546-7293, or fax 215-790-9330.

Part of the proceeds from the sale of this book will go to the Amos Christie Society at the Vanderbilt University School of Medicine.

Pearls from a Pediatric Practice ISBN 1-56053-267-X

Library of Congress Catalog Card Number 97-81436

Last digit is the print number: 9 8 7 6 5 4 3 2 1

DEDICATIONS

I dedicate this book to the
Amos Christie Society of
Vanderbilt Children's Hospital.

– WW

I dedicate this book to my children
Clifton, Aubrey, Ann, Elizabeth, Mary Kathleen,
Graham, and Rebecca
and to my wife Kathleen.

All taught and continue to teach me.

– CKM

If you would like to suggest a pearl for the next edition, please photocopy this page as many times as needed and submit to the publisher. For information about ordering bulk quantities of the book for educational purposes, contact the publisher at 215-546-7293, or fax 215-790-9330.

William Wadlington, M.D.
c/o Hanley & Belfus, Inc.
210 South 13th Street
Philadelphia, PA 19107

Pearl: ____

____

____

____

____

____

____

From (name and address): ______________________________

____

____

INTRODUCTION

It was a pleasure and privilege to work with Dr. Bill Wadlington in editing the pearls that he has gathered from his pediatric practice during the past 43 years.

I first knew Bill when he was a senior resident in pediatrics and I was a junior medical student at Vanderbilt. His ability to organize learning material and his budding propensity for generating rules and mnemonics stuck in my mind. His early influence affected my thinking when I first thought of publishing the *Little Book of Doctors' Rules*. When I was asked to publish a second volume of *Rules*, I contacted Bill. I knew he would contribute outstanding rules from his practice. As he kept sending material, it became obvious that we needed an entire book to do justice to his collection. We even included an index at the back of the book to facilitate easy access to specific pearls.

I want to thank Linda Belfus, our publisher, and Virginia Fuqua Meadows, who assisted me in the preparation of the manuscript.

Clifton K. Meador, M.D.
Nashville, Tennessee

ABOUT PEDIATRICIANS IN GENERAL
and
WILLIAM WADLINGTON IN PARTICULAR

When I was Dean of the School of Medicine at the University of Alabama in Birmingham in the late 1960s, I spent a lot of time traveling about the state. I wanted to know how we, as a state medical school, could serve the educational needs of physicians. Two groups impressed me the most: family physicians and pediatricians. I was impressed with their dedication and intensity. They were attached to their patients and the families of the patients. They knew them as people, not just as patients with some disease. They made no distinction between dysfunctions of body, mind, or spirit. The child and family were an integrated whole. They were true clinicians, calling on raw observations and keen senses about human nature. They went by what they saw, heard, felt, and even smelled. Their insistence on operating from their senses and wits made a deep impression on my clinical thinking. Bill Wadlington captures much of this spirit in the observations recorded in this book.

In the past 30 years, pediatricians have continued to be my model of the true physician. Bill Wadlington, in my opinion, is a pediatrician's pediatrician. This collection of his pearls displays his dedication to his patients, to the medical students whom he teaches every week in his office, to the community where has been so active in antismoking and other educational efforts, and to the practice of pediatrics, for which he remains an eternal student.

In 1988 Bill Wadlington was selected as Tennessee Pediatrician of the Year. In 1991 he was honored as the Tennessee Volunteer Physician of the Year. This award was given for his long efforts in working with teenagers to improve lifestyles and for his educational efforts in drug, alcohol, and tobacco abuse among children and adolescents.

At a national level he was honored twice by the American Academy of Pediatrics. In 1988 in San Francisco, he received the National Practitioner Research Award for his 36 papers about children's problems. These papers, like this book, were generated from observations in his office practice.

A second national award, the Lay Education Award of the American Academy of Pediatrics, was given in 1991 at the annual meeting in New Orleans. This award recognized his efforts in establishing the Health Hall in the Cumberland Children's Museum in Nashville. This permanent exhibit is directed at teaching children about the human body and about staying healthy.

It has been my privilege to work with Bill Wadlington in publishing these *Pearls from a Pediatric Practice*.

Clifton K. Meador, M.D.

PREFACE

In December of 1996, Dr. Clifton Meador said he was working on Volume II of his *Little Book of Doctors' Rules*. He asked me to write down a few "pediatric pearls." I gave him about 10 pages of material. He liked the writings and said, "Let's do a book."

I have tried to gear this book toward office practice (95% of all pediatrics). I have made an effort to avoid too many numbers and percentages and instead to focus on trends. In a few years someone who is much wiser will prove that some of my "pearls" are wrong. I wish I could predict which statements will stand the test of time. However, as Casey Stengel said, "Prediction is difficult, especially when it deals with the future."

Pearls from a Pediatric Practice is not intended to help students pass their board exams or to give an exhaustive list of differential diagnostic possibilities. Readers interested in such goals are referred to *The Portable Pediatrician* and *Pediatric Secrets*. This book offers a number of one-liners designed to help the pediatrician get along with patients and partners. It includes tips on managing everyday behavior problems or dispelling myths about obesity. We hope that it can be enjoyed by nonmedical people, particularly parents of young children.

Pearls are learned after years of experience and many mistakes. They are also learned from listening to physicians who have been in the trenches. This book relates some of the pearls I have learned about children and life in my 43 years of pediatric practice and 47 years of marriage.

Pearls are usually short, often dramatic, and occasionally witty. You know one when you hear it. The succinctness of pearls follows Thomas Jefferson's rule, "The most valuable of all talents is never using two words when one will do."

Quotations from a poem by Dorothy Law Nolte, "Children Learn What They Live" (1972), have been sprinkled throughout the text. I appreciate her sharing her wisdom with us. Her book, *Children Learn What They Live: Parenting to Inspire Values*, is published by Workman Publishing, New York, New York.

My scribbled notes have been typed by Mrs. Pauline Moore, who is our office manager.

Some readers may say, "That was my statement, and I made it 40 years ago!" I make no claim that these pearls are mine alone. As Osler said, "Never hide the work of others under your own name."

Finally, for the past year my family noticed the "fun" I've had writing the book. They all said they wanted to put in a "one-liner" of their own, so here goes!

Anna Wadlington (my wife)—A parent's obligation is not to make their children "happy," but to give them resources and skills to pursue happiness on their own.

Skip Bayles (my son-in-law)—Studies show that people who attend church live longer than people who don't.

Amy Bayles (Skip's wife)—After college I worked for Dr. Ken Cooper, so I believe his studies which show that 45 minutes of aerobic activity three times weekly prolongs life significantly.

Van Wadlington, M.D.—A recent study in Copenhagen found that men, on average, have about four billion more brain cells than women, but they haven't figured out what men do with them!

John Wadlington, M.D.—About thirty percent of baby boys with hemophilia have no remarkable bleeding from their circumcision procedure.

Jeff Wadlington—The "Bottom Line" (P.O. Box 58446, Boulder, CO 80322) helps me more each week than any other periodical that I read.

William Wadlington, M.D.
Nashville, Tennessee

ACKNOWLEDGMENTS

Much of my "real pediatrics" has been learned from my family: my wife (Anna), Will (who died at 10 years of age with cystic fibrosis), Amy, Van, John, and Jeff. Pediatrics was relearned with four grandchildren (Mallie, Kelly, Mazi, and Colson).

I chose pediatrics because of my mentor, Amos Christie. I had many great teachers at Vanderbilt Children's Hospital and St. Louis Children's Hospital. At present, my main teachers are the third-year medical students from Vanderbilt. My main sources of information are gleaned from the following:

1. *Audio Digest:* A subsidiary of the California Medical Association monthly tapes (1-800-423-2308). I keep at least two tapes in my car at all times.

2. *Pediatric Notes:* P.O. Box 59, Newtonville, MA 02160. The weekly comments (usually 3 pages) of Dr. Sydney Gellis and Dr. Richard Goldbloom should be carved in stone.

3. *Pediatric Annals:* Dr. Bill Altemeier has done a *great* job as editor-in-chief.

4. *Year Book of Pediatrics:* The leadership over the years of Dr. Sydney Gellis and James Stockman is unsurpassed. Dr. Stockman's comments in the articles are frequently better than the articles themselves.

5. *Contemporary Pediatrics:* I especially enjoyed the editorials by Dr. Frank Oski, who died in 1996.

6. *Instructions for Pediatric Patients:* Dr. Barton D. Schmitt offers the best instructions (hand-outs) that I have seen. They save me a *lot* of time.

7. *A Little Book of Doctors' Rules:* This book by Dr. Clifton K. Meador is filled with useful advice and is fun to read. It started me thinking that maybe I could use it as a model for a similar book called *Pearls from a Pediatric Practice.*

8. *Vanderbilt Children's Hospital:* The ward rounds and staff are unsurpassed. I am grateful to all of them.

9. Dr. H.D. Riley and Dr. Gerald Hickson reviewed the manuscript for this text and have been especially helpful. —WW

1 **Miracles at Home**

A child who can sit at a dinner table for more than 15 minutes is called a miracle.

2 **Colicky Baby**

If you want a colicky baby to sleep at night, give him or her 1 drop per pound of paregoric in about a tablespoon of milk or juice (a 10-pound baby gets 10 drops of paregoric). Then everyone can go to sleep.

3 **Rent Crutches**

Crutches are expensive to buy.

Some large grocery chains keep a supply in use.

Put down a deposit. When you return the crutches, the store returns your deposit.

4 **Nosebleeds**

- Try not to pack the nose of children who have nosebleeds.
- Teach them to apply firm pressure with a straight finger along the side of the nose.
- If you must pack the nose, a sliver of fatty bacon works well.
- When you pull out the bacon, you will not pull out the clot.

5 **Set Goals**

"No wind blows in favor of a ship without direction" (Hans Selye). You must know your goals and in what direction you are headed.

6 **Television and Video Games**

Video games may have a worse effect on the education of children than television.

7 **Treatment of Otitis Media**

- A single injection of ceftriaxone (Rocephin) is frequently as effective as 10 days of oral amoxicillin.
- Keep in mind that most children with otitis get well in spite of their doctor. Spontaneous cures are common.

8 **Parvovirus B19 Arthritis**

The arthritis caused by parvovirus B19 reminds one of the arthritis caused by rubella virus. Adults have more arthritis and less rash than children.

9 **Epidemic Sloth**

There is a national decline in physical exercise among children. Part of the decline may be due to the inactivity related to watching television.

10 **Recurrent Meningitis**

Finding the cause of recurrent meningitis is sometimes difficult:

- After checking the middle ear and lower spine for signs of fistula, look for a tiny pit on the bridge of the nose as a clue for an underlying dermoid sinus and cyst.
- A CT scan may delineate the size and course of the dermoid or sinus tract.

11 **Polycythemia and Wilms' Tumor**

- An elevated hematocrit may be a clue to an underlying Wilms' tumor of the kidney that produces erythropoietin.
- Aniridia (partial or nearly complete agenesis of the iris of one or both eyes) is another clue to a possible Wilms' tumor.

12

Television Is the Enemy

It is the most evil, insidious, unrecognized destroyer in America.

It teaches your kids the wrong values.

It destroys your muscle tone and reduces you to flab.

It eliminates social interactions (family, neighborhood, community, church, business, team, and other).

It demeans your existence by glamorizing pure poppycock.

It wastes your life with nothing to show for it.

Turn it on and enjoy a slow suicide.

From J. Clyde Ralph, M.D.
Pediatric News 1986

13 **Most Common Inherited Red Cell Disorder**

G6PD deficiency is the most common inherited disorder of the red blood cell.

14 **Echocardiography for Mitral Regurgitation**

Echocardiography can demonstrate mitral regurgitation not detectable by auscultation.

15 **Small Penis**

- A *concealed penis* is associated with an overlying fold of abdominal fat.
- A *buried penis* is a congenital anomaly that has two components: an abnormally large suprapubic fat pad plus dense fibrous bands that tether and retract the penis.
- The size of the penis is normal in both of the above. Both should be distinguished from true *micropenis*.

16 **Hypothermia and Agenesis of the Corpus Callosum**

Recurrent spontaneous hypothermia may be associated with agenesis of the corpus callosum.

17 **Malformations of the Corpus Callosum**

Agenesis (complete absence) and hypoplasia of the corpus callosum are congenital anomalies found frequently in children with mental retardation, developmental delays, infancy-onset seizures, and other congenital syndromes.

18 **Opossums Do Not Have a Corpus Callosum**

(*Editors' note:* Wadlington and Meador argued about the inclusion of this observation. Wadlington won, insisting that pediatricians have broader biologic interests than internists.)

19 **Ultrasound and Pyloric Stenosis**

Ultrasound examination is the preferred method to demonstrate or exclude the presence of pyloric stenosis.

20 **Pityriasis Rosea**

Pityriasis rosea is associated with at least two interesting particulars:

- The herald patch is often confused with ringworm (tinea corporis) before the generalized eruption appears.
- The rash never occurs above the chin or below the knees—hence the name "chin-to-knee" disease.

21 **Take Pictures in Your Office**

If bruises and burns look like child abuse, take a photograph for the chart. Keep a Polaroid camera in your office for that purpose.

22 **Jaundice in Hepatitis**

Probably 90% of children with hepatitis do not become jaundiced.

23 **Purpura**

- Below the belt: If all the purpura is below the waist (i.e., orthostatic) and the platelets are normal, think of Henoch-Schönlein purpura.
- Above the nipples: If the purpura is all above the nipples and the platelets are normal, think of Valsalva purpura associated with coughing or vomiting.

24 **Cystic Fibrosis**

The present genetic blood test for cystic fibrosis detects only 70% of cases. The other 30% represent different mutations.

25 **Shingles in Children**

Shingles in small children is not as painful as in adults.

26 **Genital Herpes**

Many episodes of primary genital herpes caused by HSV-2 are asymptomatic.

27 **Roseola and Herpesviruses 6 and 7**

Human herpesviruses 6 and 7 may cause roseola (exanthem subitum) in children. These viruses also cause sore throats, cervical adenitis, and hepatitis in children without a rash.

28 **Tuberculosis in Parent and Child**

One unusual way to diagnose tuberculosis in a parent is to find it in his or her child.

29 **Adults Do Not Whoop like Children**

- Adults with pertussis do not whoop like children.
- Pertussis is much more of an adult disease than was thought in the past.
- In outbreaks of pertussis, adults frequently get the disease and transmit it to children.

30 **Long-term Effects of Obesity**

Overweight adolescent girls, when they become women, attend school 0.3 years less, are 20% less likely to marry, and have lower household incomes and a higher rate of poverty than women who have not been overweight.

31 **Open Telephones before Office Hours**

Telephone lines should be open for appointments or advice at least one hour before the pediatrician's office opens.

If children live with criticism,
they learn to condemn.

From “Children Learn What They Live”

32 **Autistic Children**

The five most commonly reported characteristics of autism are

1. lack of awareness of others
2. impaired imitation
3. abnormal social play
4. abnormal nonverbal communication
5. absence of imaginative play

33 **Legg-Perthes Disease**

If you think a child with a limp has Legg-Perthes disease and the hip radiographs are normal, get an MRI.

34 **Arthritis with MMR Vaccine Booster**

Protracted arthritis has occurred after an injection of measles-mumps-rubella vaccine (MMR). It is thought to be associated with the rubella portion of the vaccine.

35 **Step Back and Reflect**

Whenever you have an urge to criticize, step back and use the moment as a chance for self-exploration.

36 **Hot Tub Rash**

Recurrent *Pseudomonas* folliculitis has been called "hot tub rash" or "yuppie skin disease." This infection is most common among "dinks" (double income, no kids) who spend excessive time in hot tubs or whirlpools.

37 **Myopia**

Nearsightedness is not caused by close computer work or sitting too close to the television.

38 **SIDS . . . Back Is Better**

Remember to put the baby to bed on his back to help prevent sudden infant death (SIDS).

39 **Smoking and SIDS**

Also remind mothers that SIDS is twice as common when parents smoke, especially the mother. The smoke inhaled by the baby is called passive smoking or second-hand smoke.

40 **Kawasaki and Rug Shampoos**

If you see a child with a fever of unknown origin, cervical nodes, generalized rash (with negative throat culture for streptococci) and conjunctivitis, ask about contact with shampooed carpets in the last month. These findings and history should make you think of Kawasaki syndrome.

41 **Kawasaki and Coronary Artery Aneurysms**

Intravenous immunoglobulin in a single infusion is superior to multiple daily infusions in preventing coronary artery aneurysms in Kawasaki syndrome.

42

Wadlington's C Problems

- Hypoparathyroidism

  Convulsions
  Cataracts
  Calcium (increased)
  Cutaneous defects

- Tracheoesophageal fistula

  Cough
  Choking
  Cyanosis

- Cytomegalovirus (CMV)

  Cephaly (micro and hydro)
  Cerebral **c**alcium
  Chorioretinitis
  Color (yellow and bruises)

- Types of migraine headaches

  Common
  Classic
  Complicated
  Cluster
  Confusional

- Toxoplasmosis

  Convulsions
  Chorioretinitis
  Cranial **c**alcifications

- Carnitine deficiency

  Coma (low blood sugar)
  Cardiomyopathy

Wadlington's C Problems *(Continued)*

- Lead poisoning
  Cerebrospinal fluid protein increased
  Colic
  Constipation
  Convulsions
  Coproporphyrins in urine increased

- Red Measles
  Cough
  Coryza
  Conjunctivitis

- Overdose of tricyclic drugs (especially Tofranil)
  Coma
  Cardiac arrhythmia
  Convulsions

43 **Recurrent Sinusitis**

The chief reason for treatment failure of chronic sinusitis is too short a course of antibiotic treatment. A full month of antibiotics is frequently necessary to eradicate the sinus infection.

44 **Testicular Torsion**

- Forget testicular scanning for confirmation of torsion.
- Scanning leads to needless delay and expense.
- The diagnosis is clinical.
- The treatment is immediate surgery.

45 **Rett Syndrome**

Rett syndrome is a progressive dementia in previously normal girls (always girls) with onset between the ages of 8 and 18 months. The main distinguishing feature between Rett syndrome and other syndromes with mental deficiency and seizures is the peculiar stereotypical hand-wringing movements.

46 **Back to School after Chickenpox**

Children may return to school as soon as visible lesions (face and other exposed areas) are crusting.

47 **GI Obstruction and Polyhydramnios**

Polyhydramnios may be due to high gastrointestinal obstruction in the fetus or defects in swallowing, as seen in anencephaly or other severe brain defects.

48 **Osteogenesis Imperfecta**

- Greenstick fractures are rare in osteogenesis imperfecta.
- Lower limb fractures with severe displacements are common.

49 **Black Widow Spider Bites**

The most common presenting complaints after a black widow spider bite are generalized abdominal pain and back and leg pain.

The antivenom produces a good response.

Spider bites are painful, tick bites are not.

50

Von Recklinghausen's Disease (Neurofibromatosis Type I)

According to National Institutes of Health guidelines, the patient should have two or more of the following:

1. Six or more café-au-lait spots
   - 1.5 cm or larger in postpubertal patients
   - 0.5 cm or larger in prepubertal patients
2. Two or more neurofibromata of any type or one or more plexiform neurofibroma
3. Axillary or inguinal freckling
4. Optic glioma (tumor of the optic pathway)
5. Two or more Lisch nodules (benign iris hamartoma)
6. A distinctive osseous lesion:
   - Dysplasia of the sphenoid bone
   - Dysplasia or thinning of long bone cortex
7. A first-degree relative with neurofibromatosis Type I

51 **Nasal Carriage of *Staphylococcus aureus***

Nasal carriage of *Staphylococcus aureus* may be eliminated from the nose by local applications of mupirocin ointment (Bactriban).

52 **Floppy Babies**

- In hypotonic newborns, look for drooping lids and a triangular mouth, like the opening of a pup tent. If these signs are noted, think of myotonic dystrophy.
- Then visit the mother, shake hands and observe if she can let go quickly. Does her grip "hold on"?
- Mothers with myotonic dystrophy may have premature gray hair, a pursed mouth (in contrast to the infant's triangular mouth), and an expressionless face.
- The disorder is transmitted as a dominant trait.
- Findings in the mother make the diagnosis in the infant.

53 **Microgeodic Disease**

Microgeodic disease is the name given to the punched-out lesions in the bones of toes and fingers of children with cold injuries (named after the resemblance to stone geodes).

54 **Voluntary Withholding of Stools**

Functional fecal retention with voluntary withholding of stool is by far the most common cause of constipation in childhood.

55 **Cigarette Smoking—Age of Onset**

- There is a strong correlation between the number of cigarettes smoked per day by adults with the age of onset of smoking.
- The younger the age when smoking is started, the more cigarettes smoked per day as an adult.

56 Smoking Inhibits *In Vitro* Fertilization

- There is a 30% reduction in success of *in vitro* fertilization using ova from women who are mild-to-moderate smokers.
- There is a 50% reduction in success if the woman is a moderate-to-heavy smoker.

57 More Facts about Smoking

- Fewer than 50 nonsmokers per 100,000 die of lung cancer before the age of 75 years.
- Smokers who stop smoking before the age of 30 years die at a rate of 100 per 100,000 by age 75 years.
- Smokers who wait until the age of 60 years to stop smoking die at the rate of 550 per 100,000 by age 75 years.
- Smokers who smoke all their lives die at a rate of 1,250 per 100,000 by age 75 years.

58 **Down's Syndrome**

Shortening of the humerus rather than the femur is a better ultrasound finding suggestive of Down's syndrome.

59 **Transilluminate Thyroglossal Duct Cysts**

Midline thyroglossal duct cysts do not need to be scanned. The cyst may move up when the tongue is extended. Transilluminate the cysts with a small flashlight.

60 **Genetic Diseases**

Over 3,000 diseases are known to be caused by defects in a single gene.

61 **Stiff Neck Does Not Always Mean Meningitis**

A stiff neck can be caused by meningitis but also by cervical adenitis or apical pneumonia.

62 **WBCs in the CSF With and Without Meningitis**

Observations of elevated white blood cells in the cerebrospinal fluid with otherwise normal findings and without evidence of infection of the meninges have been made in shigellosis, leptospirosis, Kawasaki disease, Behçet syndrome, and right and left upper lobe pneumonia.

- All that is meningitis need not have findings of white blood cells in the cerebrospinal fluid

  and

- All with findings of white blood cells in cerebrospinal fluid need not be meningitis.

63 **Ultrasound in Acute Surgical Abdomen**

Ultrasound studies are useful in confirming or excluding a diagnosis of acute appendicitis or ovarian cysts as the cause of the pain.

64 **Congenital Spine Abnormalities**

The presence of a patch of hair, a fistula, a pad of fat, or a nevus over the spine suggests an underlying congenital abnormality of the spine. MRI or ultrasound studies confirm or rule out the diagnosis.

65 **Alcohol Consumption in Teenagers**

- According to estimates, junior and senior high school students drink over 30 million gallons of wine coolers per year (36% of all sold) and over 1 billion cans of beer (2% of all beer sold).
- Among high school seniors, 90% report consuming alcohol at some time and 64% say they are current drinkers.
- Thirty-five percent say that they regularly get intoxicated, defined as consuming more than 5 drinks per drinking episode.

66 **Childhood Behavior Foreshadows Adult Behavior**

- Seventy-five percent of teenagers who abuse alcohol and drugs are daily cigarette smokers.
- A study of adults who abuse drugs and alcohol showed that 86% of men and 82% of women are smokers.

67 **P Antigen and Parvovirus B19**

The parvovirus binds to an antigen curiously called the P antigen, a coincidence since the P antigen was described by Landsteiner in 1928. Absence of the P antigen protects against parvovirus infection.

68 **Posterior Cervical Adenopathy**

The two most common causes of posterior adenopathy are viral infections and irritations of the back part of the scalp. (Check the scalp for chigger or tick bites in the summer.)

69

Transient Synovitis of the Hip

- Transient synovitis is the most common cause of nontraumatic limp in children 2–4 years of age.
- The child may go to bed well and wake with a limp or not wanting to walk.
- Typically the child gets better in a few days.
- The child does not need hematologic or x-ray studies on the initial visit.
- Some children have recurrences within the next few months, sometimes in the opposite limb.
- In transient synovitis of the hip, effusion is much more frequently demonstrated by ultrasound than by conventional x-ray studies.
- Close follow-up is needed to ensure that Perthes disease or some other problem is not missed.

70 Fetal Alcohol Syndrome (FAS)

- FAS is the most common cause of acquired mental retardation.
- There is no marker for past alcohol consumption in the mother. Until there is, the clinical diagnosis of FAS may be difficult.
- Characteristic facial features include a short palpebral fissure and a flat, thin upper lip. It is difficult to think of this syndrome at birth based on facial features alone.
- In infants who are small, underweight, and/or microcephalic, it is best to have a good photograph of the baby's face and a follow-up of linear growth and intellectual and social development. It sometimes requires observation of all of these elements before a diagnosis can be made, even in retrospect.

71 **Seizures and Breath-holding**

Convulsions during breath-holding spells do not indicate epilepsy and should not call for antiepileptic therapy.

72 **More about Breath-holding**

There are two types of breath-holding:

1. Breath-holding with cyanosis (blue type)
2. Breath-holding with pallor (pale type)

Anti-epileptic medications do not help with either type. Children with both types outgrow the behavior.

73 **Wilson's Disease**

Up to 15% of children with Wilson's disease who have active liver involvement may have normal ceruloplasmin levels. A negative copper stain of liver tissue does not rule out Wilson's disease. The diagnosis is clinical, requiring a combination of findings.

74 **Clinical Findings of Wilson's Disease**

- Liver disease is the primary presentation in pediatric patients, usually appearing after age five. Examples include acute hepatitis, fulminant hepatitis, chronic hepatitis, or cirrhosis.
- Neurologic symptoms appear in older children and include tremor, dysarthria, loss of fine motor control, seizures, or personality changes.

75 **Cat Scratch Fever in Girls**

There is an increased prevalence of cat scratch fever in little girls. Little girls play with kittens more than little boys do.

76 **Distance Running and Sore Nipples**

If you see a teenager with sore nipples, don't always think of infection. First, ask if the patient is a distance runner.

77 **EEGs and Petit Mal**

Absence (petit mal) seizures are the only type of epilepsy that can be diagnosed specifically by electroencephalography. The spike-and-dome, 3-per-second pattern is diagnostic.

78 **Pollakiuria—A Cause of Urgency in Parents**

- Some children urinate frequently in small amounts throughout the day and have no other urinary tract symptoms. Urine examination is normal.
- Such children probably have a condition called pollakiuria. The term comes from the Greek word *pollakes*, which means often.
- The syndrome has a sudden onset, occurs in children ages 3–5 years, appears during the waking hours only, is benign, and lasts a few weeks.
- Frequency in the child causes urgency in the parent.

79 **Munchausen and Munchausen-by-Proxy Syndromes**

- The Munchausen syndrome is present in patients who repeatedly invent outrageous stories to fool physicians.
- The Munchausen-by-proxy syndrome is child abuse in which the deceit stems from the adult, with the child as the victim.
- Be wary of the child with a history of seizures seen only by the mother. The same is true for apnea seen only by the mother.

80 **Hazards of Day Care**

Most day-care centers are the world's best incubators of bacteria and viruses.

81 **Heart Block in Newborns**

If a newborn has a heart block and the mother is not on drugs, check the mother for lupus erythematosus.

82 **Prevent Swimmer's Ear**

Swimmer's ear is usually caused by the *Pseudomonas* organism. To prevent swimmer's ear, put a few drops of rubbing alcohol into the ear canal after swimming and then gently dry the canals with a hair dryer.

83 **Swimming with Ear Tubes**

Swimming on the surface only may be permitted for a child with ear tubes (some physicians still insist on ear plugs). Under no circumstance should diving or underwater swimming be allowed.

84 **Otitis Media Is Common**

Otitis media is the most common reason (other than well baby visits) for children to be seen by health care professionals.

85 **Otitis Media: A Spectrum of Diseases**

- Acute otitis media (AOM)
- Recurrent otitis media (ROM)
- Persistent otitis media
- Otitis media with effusion (OME)
- Otitis media with drainage
- Others

86 **Risk Factors for Otitis Media**

- Smoking exposure
- Nasal allergy
- Cranial abnormalities such as cleft palate
- Prolonged bottle feedings, especially if the child is on his or her back
- Pacifiers
- History of otitis media in the parents and siblings
- Exposure to children in day care

87 **Viral Infections and Otitis Media**

Viral infections are the most common cause of otitis media. Most cases of otitis media follow an upper respiratory infection.

88 **Allergies Predispose to Otitis Media**

Allergic children have more bouts of otitis media than children who are not atopic.

89 **Frequency of Otitis Media**

- By the first birthday, nearly two-thirds of children have had one bout of acute otitis media.
- By age 3 years, almost one-half of children have had 3 or more bouts of acute otitis media.

90 **No Clubbing with Asthma**

Uncontrolled asthma does not cause clubbing.

91 **Abdominal Pain in Teenaged Girls**

Suspect hematocolpos (due to an imperforate hymen) in a teenage girl who has monthly abdominal pain but no menstrual bleeding.

92 **Turner's Syndrome (Two Types)**

- Short girls (even without neck webbing) should have chromosomal studies to rule out Turner's syndrome.
- Neck webbing is less frequent in the small ring-X chromosomal type than in the 45X type.

93 **What Pulled Elbow Is Not**

Nursemaid's elbow or pulled elbow is not the result of dislocation of the head of the radius (as taught); it is due to trapping of a synovial fold of the capsule. This was proved by repeated ultrasound studies of the elbow moved in various positions.

94 **Choosing a Partner**

Choosing a new partner in practice is like getting married. Choose carefully.

95 **Remove Smooth Foreign Bodies with a Foley Catheter**

A Foley catheter can be used to safely remove smooth foreign bodies from the esophagus.

96 **Anorexia Nervosa vs. Bulimia Nervosa**

Anorexia nervosa

- Refusal or inability to maintain body weight over a minimal normal weight
- Intense fear of gaining weight or becoming fat, despite being underweight
- Disturbance in perception of body shape
- In postmenarcheal females, absence of 3 consecutive menses

Anorexia Nervosa vs. Bulimia Nervosa *(Continued)*

Bulimia nervosa (bulimia, meaning "ox hunger," comes from Greek)

- Recurrent episodes of binge eating
- A feeling of lack of control over binge-eating behavior
- Regular use of self-induced vomiting, laxatives, diuretics, strict dieting or fasting, or vigorous exercise to prevent weight gain
- Minimum of 3 binge-eating episodes weekly for at least 3 months
- Overconcern with and disturbance in perception of body shape

97 **Diarrhea and Seizures**

If a child has diarrhea and a seizure, think shigellosis. The convulsion is due to a neurotoxin from the *Shigella* organism.

98 **Nonsteroidal Antiinflammatory Agents**

Nonsteroidal antiinflammatory agents do cause gastritis and GI ulceration in children but not nearly to the extent seen in adults.

99 **Erythema Multiforme vs. Stevens-Johnson Syndrome**

- Erythema multiforme is most often caused by herpes simplex infection.
- Stevens-Johnson syndrome is most commonly associated with drug reactions, less frequently with infections such as mycoplasma, and uncommonly with malignancies or collagen vascular diseases.

100 **Prevention of Otitis Media**

Prolonged use of pacifiers (after 9 months) and letting a baby bottle-feed on its back are two preventable causes of recurrent otitis media.

If children live with jealousy,
they learn to feel envy.

From “Children Learn What They Live”

101 **Beware of Certain Gifts**

Do not accept any gift that has to be fed.

102 **Attention Deficit Disorder (ADD) and Attention Deficit Hyperactivity Disorder (ADHD)**

- The gold standard for the diagnosis of both ADD and ADHD is <u>a history of the child's behavior</u> derived from a clinical interview and not from any test performance.
- About 5% of children in the United States are believed by some to have ADD or ADHD in one form or another.
- Their behavioral problems may be inattention, hyperactivity, or impulsive behavior over a long period.
- Any one of these three behaviors may predominate.
- About 60–70% of patients respond rapidly (within a few days) to treatment with methylphenidate (Ritalin).
- The child with a history of setting fires, harming younger children, or abusing pets needs psychiatric referral.

103 **Ritalin Dosing and Timing**

- Ritalin administration in many children may require thrice-daily doses.
- In older children a dose of 5–10 mg at 5–6 P.M. may help at homework time. It does not seem to interfere with sleep.
- Ritalin should be administered to fit the severity and timing of the problem and not in anticipation of side effects.

104 **EEGs: Limited Value to Predict Seizure Relapse**

- If a child has been seizure-free for two years, an electroencephalogram is of little value as a predictor of seizure relapse.
- If a child has been seizure-free for two years, give strong consideration to stopping anticonvulsant therapy.

105 **Fragile X Syndrome**

If you see a retarded boy with large ears and large testicles (after puberty), he has fragile X syndrome until proved otherwise.

106 **Another Tick Bite Fever: Ehrlichiosis**

- The characteristic rash is present in all children with ehrlichiosis but in only 35% of affected adults.
- Ehrlichiosis probably accounts for some cases treated as Rocky Mountain spotted fever if laboratory evidence was inconclusive.
- Chloramphenicol and tetracycline are effective treatments.

107 **Teratogenic Acne Treatment**

Accutane (for cystic acne) is the most potent teratogen currently in use.

108 **Enuresis**

If a child with nocturnal enuresis has normal voiding during the day without increased frequency, training efforts to increase bladder capacity are worthless.

109 **More about Enuresis**

- Children with enuresis are frequently sound sleepers, and there is usually a family history of bed wetting.
- If the urinalysis is normal, do not order a genitourinary tract work-up. Be patient.

110 **Intraosseous Epinephrine**

Epinephrine administered into the trachea of a child who has poor vascular access is poorly absorbed. Intraosseous administration (usually in the tibia) is more effective in such urgent situations.

111 **Punctate Epiphysis: A Sign, Not a Disease**

A punctate epiphysis is a radiologic sign and not a specific disease. There are over 20 causes for punctate or stippled epiphyses.

112 **Red Anal Area**

Marked erythema around the rectal opening may be due to beta hemolytic streptococcal infection. Use throat swabs to do a rapid streptococcal test on the red skin.

113 **Ask about Grades**

Over one-half of people who bring their children to the office do not discuss some of their main concerns (grades, poor motivation, discipline problems, and other psychosocial concerns). At the end of your examination of school-age children, always ask about the child's grades and record this information in the chart.

114 **Sinus Infections**

The most common bacterial pathogens for sinus infections are *Streptococcus pneumoniae*, *Hemophilus influenzae* (nontypable), and *Moraxella catarrhalis*. These same organisms cause bacterial otitis media.

115 **Anorectal Anomalies Associated with Spinal Cord Abnormalities**

Fifty percent of children with anorectal abnormalities (e.g., imperforate anus) have abnormalities of the spinal cord demonstrable by MRI.

116 **Excess Water Can Cause Seizures**

Inquire about excessive water drinking (especially commercial bottled water) in children with seizures. Hyponatremic seizures have been reported in over 30 children with excessive water intake.

117 **Birth Defects Are Not Increased in Gulf War Children**

At present there is no evidence of an increase in birth defects among the children of Gulf War veterans.

118 **A Lot of Diapers**

In 1991, more than 17 billion disposable diapers were sold in the United States.

119 **Down's Syndrome**

There is an increased incidence of the following conditions in Down's syndrome:

- Thyroid diseases
- Leukemia
- Celiac disease
- Duodenal atresia
- Hirschsprung's disease
- Cervical and spine abnormalities

One-half of patients with Down's syndrome have a congenital heart defect, which is usually the lesion that determines life expectancy.

120 **Fetal Cocaine and Hypertonia**

- There is a consistent association between fetal cocaine exposure and hypertonia.
- Hypertonia, consistent with cerebral palsy, diminishes over time and resolves in 97% of infants by 2 years of age.
- Arm hypertonia abates before leg hypertonia.

121 **Bee Stings and Nephrotic Syndrome**

Some children who seem to have recovered from nephrotic syndrome may promptly relapse after a bee sting. Avoid bees!

122 **Sleeping Preemies**

Warn parents that when a premature infant who previously slept peacefully comes home, crying will increase over the next 6–8 weeks.

123 **Hemophiliacs**

Hemophiliacs never present with gastrointestinal bleeding.

124 **Sources of Great Medical Tips**

Some of the best medicine tips:

- *Pediatric Notes* (monthly). Editorial comments by Dr. Sydney Gellis and Dr. Richard Goldbloom are frequently better than the articles they review.
- *Year Book of Pediatrics*. Some of the comments by Dr. James Stockman III should be carved in stone. Most of his editorials are loaded with pearls.
- *Monthly Tapes from Audio-Digest Foundation*
  California Medical Association
  1577 East Chevy Chase Drive
  PO Box 712
  Glendale, California 91209–9979
  Keep at least two tapes in your car <u>at all times</u>.

125 **Colas Do Not Cause Infections**

Drinking colas does not cause kidney infection. However, children drink too many carbonated beverages, said to average 30 gallons a year.

126 **Babies with Pneumonia Breathe Fast**

An infant under 1 year of age with a respiratory rate less than 50 per minute is highly unlikely to have pneumonia.

127 **Baby Smiles**

Watch a 5-month-old baby smile. Everyone who sees him or her immediately smiles. Learn from babies.

128 **Be Wary of Ordering Chest X-Rays in Small Children**

Radiologic findings on chest radiographs in small children appear to be poor indicators of an etiologic diagnosis.

129 **Asthma and Cigarette Smoking**

- There is a significant correlation between the number of cigarettes smoked in the house and indicators of asthma severity.
- Children of mothers who smoke are more severely affected in the cold, wet season than in the warm, dry season.

130 **Partners Need Support**

When you see one of your partner's patients, put in a good word for your partner:

- "He does a good job, doesn't he?"
- That was a good diagnosis she made."
- "She is dependable, isn't she?"

You will feel good and your partner will feel great when he or she hears about it. We all need encouragement from time to time.

131 **Botulinum Toxin as a Treatment**

There are an increasing number of indications for treatment of various conditions with botulinum toxin:

- Masseter muscle hypertrophy
- Various types of cervical dystonia
- Blepharospasm
- Spasmodic dysphonia
- Strabismus
- Spasticity in cerebral palsy
- Familial chin trembling
- Painful anal sphincter spasm

132 **Time Is Measured in Minutes in Treating Meningitis**

If you have a child with a petechial rash and you are worried about meningococcal infection, treat them *immediately*, while your nurse calls the emergency department.

133 **Amblyopia**

- Amblyopia is the most frequent cause of impaired vision in children and young adults.
- Caretakers of children need to do thorough visual examinations starting at age 3 years.
- Always ask about a family history of "lazy eye."

134 **Oligohydramnios**

Oligohydramnios may be a clue to a renal problem in the fetus.

135 **Diet and the Causes of Death**

Of the 10 leading causes of death in the United States, five have proven links to diet:

- Heart disease
- Stroke
- Diabetes mellitus
- Atherosclerosis
- Certain cancers

136 **Use Inexpensive Eyedrops**

Because it is difficult at times to distinguish bacterial from viral conjunctivitis, use eyedrops Medicaid will pay for (garamycin).

137 **Hospital Admissions**

- Utilization studies show that one-fourth of pediatric hospitalizations are unnecessary.
- Results in Canada, which has a different insurance and health system, are not very different.
- As you gain more experience, you hospitalize fewer patients.

138 **Skin Lubricant**

If a parent insists on lubricating a child's dry skin, Mazola cooking oil works about as well as anything—and it's cheap.

139 **Popliteal Artery Entrapment**

If a child has acute or insidious onset of pain in the leg below the knee with radiation to the foot, think of popliteal artery entrapment syndrome. This rare syndrome is mentioned only because the surgical treatment may be simple and curative (like clipping a fibrous band).

140 **Idiopathic Hypercalciuria**

- There are two subtypes: absorptive and renal.
- The diagnosis requires 24-hour urine measurements of calcium and sodium, combined with calcium loading and deprivation.
- Think of this diagnosis in any child with nephrolithiasis, enuresis, hematuria, or colicky abdominal pain.
- These symptoms and findings may occur singly or in combination.

141 **Retropharyngeal Swelling: Abscess or Cellulitis?**

If you need help with the early management of a possible retropharyngeal abscess, ultrasound of the neck may help to distinguish the swollen nodes of cellulitis from an abscess. Children with abscesses usually hyperextend their necks. If you still are not sure, get a good ear-nose-throat surgeon.

142 **Cerebral Palsy**

Most cases of cerebral palsy are related to problems in fetal development and <u>not to the lack of skills or neglect of the obstetrician</u>.

143 **A Rash Is Worth a Thousand Words**

Erythema migrans is pathognomonic of Lyme disease. The rash, if present, is more valuable diagnostically than any laboratory test.

144 **Williams Syndrome**

Williams syndrome is a developmental disorder characterized by a unique facial appearance with a large mouth and prominent lips, supravalvular aortic stenosis, and hypercalcemia.

145 **Predictors of Future Febrile Seizures**

Several factors are predictive of future seizures after a first febrile seizure.

- Family history of febrile seizures in a first- or second-degree relative
- Increased viral exposure (e.g., child in day care)
- Long length of stay in a neonatal unit
- Slow development
- Very low birth weight

The more of these factors present, the higher the likelihood of recurrent febrile seizures.

146 **Febrile Seizures and Anticonvulsants**

Which children with febrile seizures need anticonvulsants later?

- Prolonged febrile seizure over 30 minutes
- Febrile seizure with focal signs
- Positive family history of seizures in parent or close relative
- Abnormal electroencephalogram a few weeks after the seizure
- Seizure with a low fever of 101° F or less

147 **Prophylactic Corticosteroids**

Prophylactic corticosteroids are helpful in preventing postextubation stridor and respiratory distress in preterm, high-risk infants. They are also useful when used early in the treatment of croup and asthma. Always use them for these indications.

148 **Five Tick Bite Diseases**

- Rocky Mountain spotted fever
- Lyme disease
- Babesiosis (in asplenic patients)
- Ehrlichiosis
- Tick paralysis

149 **Dogs Have Their Own Lice**

Lice are host-specific. Dog lice will not parasitize humans. Human lice do not parasitize dogs.

150 **Child Treatment vs. Stool Treatment**

Most children with acute diarrhea can be managed with continued feedings of undiluted nonhuman milk. Lactose-free formulas appear to be of limited value. Let them have small amounts of solids if they so desire.

Treat the child, not the stool!

151 **Reflex Sympathetic Dystrophy**

Pain and striking sensitivity of a limb in the absence of trauma or infection in a child should suggest reflex neurosympathetic dystrophy (RSD).

152 **Recurrent Parotid Swelling**

There are several causes of recurrent parotid swelling:

- Sjögren's syndrome (dry mouth, positive biopsy, positive antinuclear antibodies)
- Benign recurring parotitis
- Congenital anomalies
- Infections (viral and bacterial)
- Air blown up Stensen's duct
  - Blowing musical instruments
  - Self-induced
  - Blowing up balloons
- Allergy to certain foods

153 **Some Things Are Not Getting Better**

We are doing a good job of controlling diseases with new drugs, better vaccines and more high-tech machines. We need improvement in the areas of helping patients with lifestyle problems:

- Drug excesses (alcohol, tobacco, street drugs)
- Food excesses (25% of teenagers are obese)
- Television excesses (children watch 4–5 hours/day)
- Violent behavior
- Too little exercise
- Decrease in respect for authority (teachers, police officers)
- Divorce rate of 50%
- School drop-out rates in excess of 20% in many public inner city schools

154 **Syncytial Virus and Otitis Media**

Acute otitis media develops in about one-third of children with respiratory syncytial virus (RSV).

155 **Read Dr. Barton Schmitt**

If you want good advice or hand-out sheets for parents, use Dr. Barton Schmitt's book, *Instructions for Pediatric Patients*. His advice is superb.

156 **Megalencephaly vs. Macrocephaly**

- If most of the family members have big heads, this is called megalencephaly. It is frequently familial and the term is intended to mean a large brain with ventricles of appropriate size.
- Macrocephaly is more common and indicates a large cranium that may or may not have underlying pathology.

157 **Delay of Cord Separation**

At least three factors are known to be involved:

- Failure of normal function of neutrophils
- Inadequate number of neutrophils
- Application of triple dye to the umbilicus

158 **Pertussis vs. Mycoplasma**

Many coughing patients with pertussis have chest x-rays that do not show pneumonia. However, many coughing patients with mycoplasmal infections show pneumonia on chest x-ray. The isolation of either organism may prove difficult.

159 **Mothers Know a Lot about Babies**

If a woman has five or more children, see what pearls you can learn from her. She does not need much advice about babies from you.

160 **Chronic Abdominal Pain**

When you are trying to determine the cause of chronic abdominal pain in children, have the parent keep a careful diary:

- What did the child do that day?
- When was the last bowel movement?
- What was eaten?
- How much?
- Don't just say pizza; put down what kind, what topping, any special sauces.

161 **Stool Cultures in the Office**

The typical rate of recovery of pathogens from routine bacterial stool cultures in most laboratories is less than 10%. There is no need to get a stool culture in the office unless the child looks sick or there is blood in the stool exam.

162 Parvovirus B19 and Fetal Hydrops

- The first proved fetal death due to parvovirus B19 was in 1984.
- Now the parvovirus B19 is the most common cause of nonimmune fetal hydrops.
- The anemia (not the myocarditis) appears to be the main culprit. A number of babies have been saved by intrauterine transfusions.
- Most infected pregnant women have no rash and show few signs of parvovirus B19 infection.

163 Isolated Findings of Puberty

The finding of isolated pubic hair or isolated breast development without advanced bone age or growth spurt often represents premature adrenarche or thelarche, benign disorders that do not require treatment.

164 **Management of Intussusception**
If you suspect the diagnosis of intussusception, confirm its presence with an ultrasound examination. This is a reasonable course of management:

- With a pediatric surgeon present, try to reduce the mass with air or saline.
- If it reduces, follow the child closely.
- If it does not reduce, turn the case over to the consulting surgeon.

165 **Ritalin Prescriptions Increasing**
About 6 million prescriptions for Ritalin (methylphenidate) were filled in 1996.

166 **C.S. Lewis**
"Prayer doesn't change God. It changes me." Maybe doctors need to use the power of prayer more.

167 **Fat Globules in Hemarthrosis**

If you aspirate blood from a joint, set some of it aside. Later, it you see fat globules on top of the blood, the patient has interarticular fracture.

168 **Osteomyelitis in Premature Infants**

- In a premature baby, remember that the earliest sign of osteomyelitis may be lack of motion of an arm or leg.
- If you suspect osteomyelitis, aspirate the affected area early.
- Do not wait for fever, increased white count, x-ray changes.
- A negative aspiration is great news!

169 **Red Stools**

Everything that is red in the stool of children is not blood. Check it out.

170 **Rectal Polyps**

Rectal polyps are almost unknown under 2 years of age. Bleeding from rectal polyps is usually painless.

171 **Anal Fissures**

Most anal fissures that cause bleeding are located at 6 and 12 o'clock.

172 **Simple Guide for Fractures**

The patient who refuses to bear weight on a foot or leg after an injury has a fracture until proved otherwise. Always ask if the patient heard a "snap" or "pop."

173 **Wash Hands**

"Laying on of hands" is important. But remember, it is the most common method of laying on pathogens. Wash hands between patients.

174 **There is a Time for "Time in" and a Time for "Time out"**
For every time-out, there ought to be a couple of time-ins, when parents spend thoughtful, peaceful time with their child.

175 **Cracked Nipples**
If a breast-feeding child has blood in the stool the first 2–3 days of life, check to see if the mom has cracked nipples.

176 **Eyedrops**
Do not fight a child to put in eyedrops. Put the drops in while the child is asleep.

177 **Spare the Medicines**
A good pediatrician uses medicines sparingly. Probably 85% of pediatric infections are viral.

178 **Document Everything**

Judges and juries consider information in the medical record to carry great weight, usually greater than the testimony of the patient-turned-plaintiff.

179 **Coronary Aneurysms in Kawasaki's Disease**

- The size of coronary aneurysms at the time of diagnosing Kawasaki's disease has been an important prognostic indicator.
- Complete resolution occurs with most aneurysms less than 4 mm in diameter.
- Aneurysms with a diameter of 4–8 mm tend to regress with rare long-term sequelae.
- Giant coronary aneurysms, with a diameter greater than 8 mm, often persist or become obstructive with the development of thromboses or stenoses.

180 ***H. pylori* Infections**

- All patients who have *Helicobacter pylori* infection have gastritis (even without symptoms).
- Histologic examination of gastric biopsy for the presence of *H. pylori* is the most sensitive and specific technique available to make the diagnosis.
- Culture of *H. pylori* is difficult and does not play much of a role in diagnosis.
- Perhaps that is why the organism was missed for so long.

181 **Watch Out for the "Black Box Areas" in the PDR**

If you ignore the statements in the "black box area" of the *Physicians' Desk Reference*, you will lose your lawsuit.

182 **Giardiasis**

Giardiasis is probably the most common parasitic cause for diarrhea in the developed world.

183 **Ask the Right Question in the Right Way**

If you do not ask the right question in the right way, you may not get the right answer.

184 **Rephrase Important Questions**

Because the history is the most important diagnostic tool in pediatrics, ask the same important question in at least two or three different ways.

185 **Myths about Breast-feeding**

Myth: Breast-feeding should be discontinued if the infant fails to thrive.

Myth: The mother's milk is not rich enough.

Myth: The mother is unable to make enough milk. If she wants to continue breast-feeding, she must supplement with formula.

If children live with sharing,
they learn generosity.

From "Children Learn What They Live"

186 **Worries of Parents and Their Children**

- *Parents' major concerns* for their children include bicycle and car accidents, head injuries, abduction, exposure to environmental poisons, appropriate discipline, values and morals, affection, finances, too much television, and eating promptly.
- *School children's concerns* differ from their parents'.
- *Boys' concerns:* having to eat food they do not like, finances, failure, and criticism.
- *Girls' concerns:* dangers of abduction, burglars, strange people following them, and death.
- *Both sexes* worry about looking foolish, people telling lies about them, being in a big crowd, and failing tests.

187 **Laughing Is Contagious**

Remind yourself to laugh more. It will be contagious for your children.

188 **Neurocysticercosis**

Neurocysticercosis, caused by the tapeworm *Taenia solium*, is the most common parasitic disease of the central nervous system.

189 ***Pneumocystis carinii***

Pneumocystis carinii is the parasitic organism most commonly associated with respiratory illness in immunocompromised patients.

190 **Common Causes of Bacterial Enteritis**

Salmonella, *Shigella*, and *Campylobacter* species are the most common causes of acute bacterial enteritis in the United States.

191 **Staphylococcal Food Poisoning**

Staphylococcus aureus is the most common cause of toxin-related food poisoning in the United States.

192 **Oxygen in Near Drowning**

The single most important therapeutic intervention in treating a near-drowning victim is the use of supplemental oxygen.

193 **Trauma: Number-one Killer**

More than 22,000 children between the ages of 1 and 19 years die each year from trauma. Brain injury is the leading cause of death.

194 **Residents Need to Visit a Pediatric Office**

When you are a resident, a few weeks in a good pediatric office is the way to learn what you need to know about pediatric practice. Less than 5% of your income will come from hospital practice. When you finish residency, will you know how to remove warts?

195 **Eosinophilia in FUO**

The presence of eosinophilia in a patient with fever of unknown origin (FUO) should alert the clinician to the possibility of a helminth infestation.

196 **Sustained Eosinophilia**

Sustained high-grade eosinophilia is unusual and typically seen only during active infestation with visceral larva migrans or trichinosis, which remain in the tissue throughout their life cycles. Children with visceral larva migrans are frequently <u>dirt eaters</u>.

197 **Tattoos and Attitude**

You cannot tell a woman with a tattoo very much. This is especially true if the tattoo is a large reptilian form (like a dragon with flames coming out of the mouth) on an exposed body part.

198 **Red Flags for Suicides**

- Recent loss of a family member
- Exposure to suicide
- Prior attempts
- Suicidal ideation
- Physical illness or injury
- Intense life stresses
- Poor coping
- Social isolation
- Family history of affective disorders
- Interpersonal problems with peers
- Sexual identity concerns
- Abuse or neglect

199 **Beckwith-Wiedemann Syndrome**

If a newborn has a large protruding tongue and a normal thyroxine blood level (T4), think of Beckwith-Wiedemann syndrome. A newborn with this syndrome has macroglossia, omphalocele, large body size, hot cross bun markings on the ear lobes, and large viscera. Watch for hypoglycemia.

200 **Parents Teach about Drugs**
When parents stop smoking, they give their children a great lesson about drugs.

201 **Don't Use Only 911**
Don't rely solely on 911 if your child has an emergency. Also have by your phone the direct numbers of your police precinct, emergency room, and firehouse.

202 **Define Problems Accurately**
If you do not correctly define the problem that exists, you may waste a lot of time trying to solve problems that do not exist.

203 **Stop Smoking for Two Weeks**
If a patient stays off cigarettes for 2 weeks, he or she has a 50% chance of succeeding for 1 year.

204 **Hot Water from the Faucet**

When you make the baby's formula, run in warm water from the faucet. Then you do not have to heat the bottle. Never heat the milk bottle in the microwave.

205 **Insomnia**

Antidepressants are not habit-forming and are better suited for long-term use to treat insomnia than hypnotic-sedatives.

206 **Panic Disorders—New Treatment**

In 1996 the Food and Drug Administration approved paroxetine (Paxil) for the treatment of panic disorders and obsessive compulsive disorders. Previously approved for the treatment of depression, paroxetine is now the first selective serotonin reuptake inhibitor (SSRI) to be approved for panic disorder.

207 **Be Careful What You Look For**

Do not look for something that you do not know what to do with if you find it.

208 **Inherited Causes of Hypercoagulability**

- Protein C deficiency
- Protein S deficiency
- Antithrombin III deficiency
- Heparin cofactor II deficiency
- Dysfibrinogenemia
- Homocystinuria
- Hypoplasminogenemia
- Activated protein C resistance

209 **Foods that Cause Anaphylaxis**

- Eggs
- Fish
- Milk
- Peanuts
- Shellfish (clams, crab, lobster, oyster, shrimp)
- Tree nuts (almonds, Brazil nuts, cashews, filberts, pecans, walnuts)

210 **Septic Joint? Aspirate**

When you are considering aspiration for a suspected septic joint, do it. Blood cultures reveal an organism in only 70–80% of patients with septic joints.

211 **Activated Charcoal Does Not Work for the Following Ingested Materials**

- Alcohols and glycols (methanol, ethanol, isopropyl alcohol)
- Petroleum distillate hydrocarbons
- Caustic agents
- Iron
- Lead
- Lithium
- Mercury
- Arsenic
- Rapid-onset agents such as cyanide or strychnine

212 **Make Learning Fun**

Help children to see how much fun it is to learn something new.

213 **Wadlington P Problems**

- White blood cell count over 20,000

Pyelitis
Pneumonia
Pertussis
Purulent infections (meningitis, abdominal abscess, etc.)

- Lupus erythematosus

Patches
Photosensitivity
Pharyngeal ulcers
alo**p**ecia*
Pain (arthritis, myositis, serositis)
Positive antinuclear antibody and Coombs' test
Pleuritis
Pericarditis
Proteinuria
Psychosis (and convulsions)
Penia (white blood cells and platelets)
Pallor (hemolytic anemia)

* A bit of a stretch!

Wadlington P Problems (*Continued*)

- Diabetes Mellitus
  Polyuria
  Polydipsia
  Polyphagia
  Pruritus

- Glioma
  Pain (eye)
  Papilledema
  Proptosis

- Porphyria
  Photosensitivity
  Pressure (B.P. increased)
  Pain (abdominal)
  Peripheral neuritis
  Psychosis
  Pallor (if anemia present)
  Pigmentation
  Porphobilinogen (urine)

214 **Ask about School Grades**

Asking and recording a child's school grades is an essential part of the history. Do so annually. Falling grades may be an early sign of emotional problems or drug usage or family discord.

215 **Climbing Out of Cribs**

If a toddler is climbing out of the crib, let him or her sleep in shoes with the laces tied loosely together. The child can still stand and walk but cannot climb!

216 **Keep a Notebook**

Keep an "interesting patient" notebook. You will be glad you did. Occasionally you may want to look up a patient you saw 20–30 years ago and get a follow-up.

217 **Most Common Cause of Sudden Cardiac Death in Young Athletes**

The most common cause of sudden cardiac death in young athletes is hypertrophic cardiomyopathy. It is usually familial. Although there is yet no cure, advice about lifestyle and drugs such as beta blockers and calcium channel blockers is helpful.

218 **Smokers Get in Trouble**

A teenager who smokes is frequently a poor student who is headed for trouble.

219 **Fever and White Counts**

- A 6-month-old girl with a fever of 104° who does not look very sick and has a white count of 5,000 probably has a viral illness.
- A 6-month-old girl with a fever of 104° who does not look very sick and has a white count of over 20,000 has a urinary tract infection until proved otherwise. Tape a plastic bag on her quickly.

220 **Compliment Good Parents**

Tell parents they are doing a great job (if they are). They frequently need the encouragement. You will see a big smile.

221 **Magic Can Be Magic**
Learn a few magic tricks to do for children. During the next visit they will ask to see another trick from the "magic" doctor.

222 **Simple Explanations**
- When explaining an illness to a patient or parent, use as many pictures as possible.
- Tell them what to expect.
- Do not use big medical words.
- Tell them "bad diseases" that they do not have (e.g., pneumonia, cancer).

223 **Nantucket Knees, Bell's Palsy, and Lyme Disease**
Any child with arthritis of the knees (known as Nantucket knees) and Bell's palsy has Lyme disease until proved otherwise.

224 **Otitis Media and Antibiotics**

If two different antibiotics do not work in a child with otitis media, a third antibiotic probably will not help. (Remember, you usually don't know what organism you are treating.) Try reviewing basic principles (e.g., nasal aspiration, saline nose drops, no pacifier) and work on better eustachian drainage.

225 **Limited Value for Chest X-rays**

In children, chest x-rays on the first day or two of a febrile illness are rarely helpful.

226 **Scratching Children**

To keep a child from scratching at night, pull the pajama sleeves over the hands and tie the sleeves. This works better than gloves. The same strategy works for thumb-sucking.

227 **Tobacco, Pot, and Cocaine**

If a teenager smokes tobacco, the chance of smoking pot increases 100-fold and the chances of using cocaine increases 30-fold.

228 **Acute Appendicitis in Children**

- Acute appendicitis <u>does not start with fever</u>.
- The child almost always vomits at least once and has anorexia.
- You will be surprised how often a family history of appendicitis is present.
- If the child walks "bent over," watch out!

229 **Children Smokers Become Adult Smokers**

Smoking is a major pediatric problem. It is a lethal adult problem. Ninety percent of adults who smoke started smoking before the age of 18 years.

230 **Eyestrain**

Eyestrain does not cause severe headaches in children.

231 **Injections vs. Oral Medicine**

Injections cannot be spilled, refused at home, vomited, forgotten, left unfilled, or poorly absorbed by the GI tract. Finally, most parents prefer an injection.

232 **Put Journal Articles in the Chart**

In patients with rare diseases or complicated medical problems, put relevant journal articles in their charts. Several purposes are served:

- The family knows you are keeping up on the latest material.
- It shows you care.
- You get a brief refresher review of the literature with each visit.

233 **Put Newspaper Clippings in the Chart**

If your patient or his or her family is in the newspaper, clip out the article and put it in the record. Do the same with Christmas cards or holiday cards or thank-you notes, yours and theirs.

234 **Print Common Prescriptions**

Have your common prescriptions preprinted. It will save you time. The pharmacist will be able to read them.

235 **Use Safe Placebos**

If you use placebos, choose one that is safe and has no side effects.

236 **Families Teach Us**

Learn something from every family you meet. All are interesting.

237 **Get Pharmacists to Call You**

- Save yourself time with patient telephone calls.
- Do not call in prescriptions to pharmacies.
- Ask your patients to have the pharmacist call your office.
- Leave your notes and orders with your nurse.

238 **Time Is a Great Healer**

Most children get well in spite of what you do. Be patient.

239 **Meet with Your Partners and Staff**

- Meet with your partners and office staff on a regular basis.
- Take minutes.
- Give a copy of the agenda to each person at the meeting.
- It is wise to have your decisions and agreements in writing for the future.

240 **Read about Your Patients**

Try to read about your patient's disease the same day that you see the patient.

241 **Cats vs. Dogs**

- Cats cause more allergy problems than dogs.
- Cats lick their fur more than dogs.
- Dried cat saliva is a frequent allergen.

242 **Progress Notes on Following Moles**

To follow the size of a mole, trace it on transparent paper. Paste the tracing on the chart.

243 **Otitis Media and Hearing Checks**

If a child has otitis media, check the hearing of both ears in the office. Hearing loss is something to follow. Teach the parent how to do this.

244 **Cute Babies**

Nearly all babies are cute. Let the parents know that.

245 **Visit Other Offices**

When you start practice, visit as many physician offices as you can. You will learn some things to do and many things not to do.

246 **Normal Growth Rules Out a Lot**

Normal progressive growth, plotted on a growth chart, is excellent evidence against chronic organic disease.

247 **Call and Check after Hospitalization**

After a patient goes home from the hospital, develop a routine of calling in a few days to see how the patient is doing. This practice is helpful with newborns. Parents will be grateful, and you will avoid many mistakes.

248 **Happiness Is a Choice**

Most people can be as happy as they want to be. It is largely a choice. Choose to make it a good day.

249 **Know When to Sit Tight**

- If a patient is getting better, do not order more lab tests.
- If the patient is getting worse, do something different.
- As they say in poker, "Hold them or fold them."

250 **Apologize When You Are Late**

When you are running late, apologize when you enter the room with the patient. Let the patient or parent know that you realize their time is valuable.

251 **Bacterial Pneumonia and Blood Cultures**

Seventy percent of children with bacterial pneumonia do not have a positive blood culture.

252 **Dizziness: An Early Symptom of Migraine**

Intermittent dizziness in a child with no other findings may be the first symptom of migraine. Because migraine can be transmitted as autosomal dominant trait, ask about a family history of migraine.

253 **Tobacco: A Deadly Vice**

Annual deaths (430,000 per year) attributed to tobacco use are greater than the total combined deaths caused by AIDS, automobile accidents, alcohol, suicide, homicide, fires, and illegal drugs. Prevention of nicotine addiction in childhood should be a national and pediatric priority.

254 **Too Many Drugs**

The more drugs a patient is taking, the harder it is to predict how they will interact and the greater the risk of complications.

255 **For Residents in Training**

- Carry self-addressed stamped postcards in your pocket.
- When a patient is discharged from the hospital, tell the patient and family, "I have enjoyed helping with the care of your child. Would you please write me in a couple of weeks on this card and let me know about your child's progress?"
- You will be surprised how much you learn about the courses of disease and how appreciated you will feel when you get the responses.

256 **Tylenol and Codeine**

Tylenol with codeine is a good drug for any parent to have available. With a small child screaming at 2 A.M., no parent can find out which ear is hurting or, for that matter, if the ear is hurting at all. *Ear drops do not help colic!*

257 **Rough Skin**

Scarlet fever in black people cannot be seen. Called "rough skin," the rash can be palpated.

258 **PACES for Teenagers**

Try putting your teenagers through PACES.

- Ask what they wish to be when they grow up, what their goals are, and how they are doing in school. Say, "Now that takes care of E for education." Then circle the E.
- Then say, "Let's talk about C for cigarettes."
- Then discuss P for pot and A for alcohol.
- They will guess that S is for sex before you get to it.

With parents out of the room, teenagers often open up and become amazingly honest. If any of the categories is a real or potential problem, capitalize the letter (paCes for example) as a reminder for the next visit.

259 **Parents Have First Names, Too**

When appropriate, call parents by their first names.

260 **Polydactyly**

The finding of five digits at the time of your examination does not rule out polydactyly, an important finding to suggest several congenital syndromes. Ask about removal of a digit or look for small scars of excisions, if clinically warranted.

261 **Method to Follow Hand Muscle Strength**

For patients with known or suspected neuromuscular diseases or arthritis:

- Roll up a blood pressure cuff and tape it at around 20 mm.
- Have patients squeeze as hard as they can.
- Record the highest pressure achieved.
- Progress or regression can be documented.

262 **The A's of Sudden Death**

- Abuse
- Asphyxia
- Aspiration
- Anaphylaxis
- Agammaglobulinemia
- Arrhythmia

263 **Difficult Families**

With a noncompliant and difficult family (known not to follow instructions or rarely to keep return appointments), change your terminology to make the condition sound its worst. Say:

- "Double pneumonia" rather than "walking pneumonia."
- Scarlet fever rather than strep throat with a rash.
- Rupture rather than hernia, if you are urging repair.

264 **Crohn's Disease and Growth Curves**

With a teenager who has occasional abdominal pain and who "falls off" the growth curve, think Crohn's disease.

265 **Obesity: A Big Problem**

Obesity in children is common (at least 20% of school-aged children). Reduce the amount of television and calories. Increase the amount of exercise.

266 **Fever and Increased Respiratory Rate**

Increased respiratory rate is a useful clinical sign of pneumonia. Fever itself elevates the respiratory rate. How much? For each degree centigrade of temperature above normal, subtract 3.7 breaths per minute.

267 **Be Cautious**

Approach the following situations carefully:

- A naked male baby
- A worn-out, sleepless mom who has a baby with colic
- A 2-year-old eating red, sticky candy
- A 3-year-old wearing cowboy boots

268 **Helicopter Mothers Switch to Velcro**

Helicopter mothers who "hover over" their young children become Velcro™ mothers who cannot let go of their teenagers later in life.

269 **Don't Worry Parents about Functional Murmurs**

- When you hear what you believe is a functional murmur, record it in the chart.
- Do not tell the parent, "I hear a heart murmur, but don't worry about it."
- Parents remember being told of any murmur for years.
- There is no need to introduce more parental anxiety into the rearing of children.

270 **Cat Scratch Fever**

An isolated enlarged lymph node should suggest cat scratch disease. Inquire about cats, especially kittens.

271 **Lumbar Puncture Resistance**

If it takes at least three nurses to hold a child for a lumbar puncture, the child probably does not have meningitis.

272 **A Picture Is Worth a Thousand Words**

Direct observation of a seizure is very helpful. Occasionally a parent will have enough presence of mind to videotape the seizure.

273 **Some Swollen Parotids Are Full of Air**

- All swollen parotid glands are not mumps.
- A swollen parotid with crepitation (palpable free air under the skin) indicates that air has been blown into Stensen's duct.
- Inquire about blowing balloons or musical instruments.

274 **Removal of a Bug from the Ear Canal**

- Take the patient into a dark room.
- Shine a light into the ear.
- The bug will come to the light.
- If the bug does not come out, flush it out.

275 **Continuity of Friendships**

Not until age 7 or 8 does a child develop a sense of continuity with a friend.

276 **Head Size May Be Determined before Birth**

- A small or large head at birth may indicate brain disease that occurred before birth.
- Take careful head measurements in all newborn infants.
- Your measurements will be invaluable for obstetric colleagues even years later.

277 **Murmurs and Coarctation of the Aorta**

When you hear a murmur in a small child, always palpate the femoral pulse to rule out coarctation of the aorta.

278 **The Parents' Guide**

One of the best books for solutions to common behavioral problems in the home is entitled *The Parents' Guide* by Stephen McCarney and Angel Bauer (Publisher Hawthorne Educational Services, 800 Gray Oak Drive, Columbia, Ohio 65201).

279 **Exudates Are Not Much Help**

The presence of an exudate does not help with the clinical diagnosis of strep throat. Many viruses can cause exudates on the tonsils. A good example is mononucleosis. A throat culture for group A streptococci is rarely indicated in patients under the age of 3–4 years.

280 **Injectable vs. Oral Methotrexate**

A teenager with rheumatoid arthritis had a cost-saving tip. He said that his oral methotrexate cost $55.00 per month. He is now giving his own injections of methotrexate (weekly) at a cost of $10.00 per month.

281 **Nosebleeds and Allergy**

Nasal allergy is the most common cause of nosebleeds.

282 **Smoking and ADHD**

Smoking may be both a cause and effect of attention deficit hyperactivity disorder (ADHD). Of 140 children with ADHD, 80% had mothers who smoked during pregnancy compared with 40% of 120 children without ADHD. Of children with ADHD, 20% were smokers during adolescence compared with only 10% of the children without ADHD.

283 **Washing Ear Wax**

Tired of washing ear wax with a syringe? A dental water pic squirts a good stream of water and makes the job easier.

284 **Cat Scratch Fever without a Cat Scratch**

Cat scratch fever may occur without a known scratch of a cat. The inoculation site may be the conjunctiva with resultant preauricular adenitis and conjunctivitis, called oculoglandular syndrome.

285 **Treat for Giardiasis**

If you have a previously well child who develops chronic diarrhea, treat the child for giardiasis. There is no need to fool with a lot of stool exams if you are going to treat for giardiasis anyway (especially if there is some evidence for malabsorption and the patient is a camper or in day care).

286 **Doing Better with Cancer, Not So Good with Guns**

- According to a California study, the 5-year survival rate of children under 20 for all cancers increased from 55% in 1974–1976 to 70% in 1986–1991.
- Survival with leukemia rose from 44% to 70% and survival with non-Hodgkin's lymphomas from 44% to 69%.
- We are doing a lot better with cancer deaths than we are with handgun and car accident deaths.

287 **Take Telephone Numbers on Trips**

Carry a home telephone book with you on trips.

288 **Confidentiality for Teenagers**

Discussing confidentiality makes teenagers more likely to talk about sexual behaviors, substance abuse, and emotional problems.

289 **Know What Symptoms Are Not Streptococcal**

- Streptococci <u>do not cause</u> rhinitis, laryngitis, bronchitis, and certainly not diarrhea.
- A runny nose, hoarseness, and cough are symptoms of a viral infection, not of streptococcal pharyngitis.

290 **Office Photography**

If you have good medical photographs, you should submit them to *Consultant Magazine*, Cliggott Publishing Company. The magazine pays $50.00 for each photo that it uses.

291 **Keep Family Memories**

Make scrapbooks about your family, relatives, and friends. They are great fun to review every few years. Have your children make scrapbooks when they return from vacations.

292 **Preparation of Children for Surgery**
There is no need to restrict oral liquids until 2 hours before most surgical procedures.

293 **Fifth Disease**
Red cheeks in a child who does not look ill and has a lacy red rash on the abdomen and limbs is highly suggestive of "fifth disease" (erythema infectiosum).

294 **Rash Means that Parvovirus B-19 Infection Is Safe**
When the rash of parvovirus B-19 infection appears on patients, *they are no longer contagious*. A lot of school teachers do not know this.

295 **Home Alone**
Teach your children never to tell anyone that they are home alone.

296 **Explaining Death to a Child**

The most important part of any explanation of death to a child is reassurance. Although the death of a loved one creates a void in a child's life, make sure that the child understands that he or she will not be alone. Telling the child, "No matter what happens, there will always be someone here to take care of you," accompanied by plenty of reassuring hugs, is the kind of comforting response needed.

297 **Sepsis vs. Respiratory Distress Syndrome in Neonates**

In neonates, it is frequently difficult to tell the difference between respiratory distress syndrome of prematurity and early-onset group B streptococcal sepsis with pneumonia. Septic babies are more likely to have hypotension but as a late finding. The first finding is tachycardia.

298 **Chickenpox Vaccine**

In 1955 the average American child missed 8.7 days of school and the average adult up to 1.8 days of work outside the home because of chickenpox. With the varicella vaccine, this disease should disappear in time.

299 **Fence in Swimming Pools**

If you have a swimming pool, it should be surrounded by a fence 4–5 feet high. The fence should have a self-locking gate that automatically swings shut.

300 **Rectal Sparing: Uncommon in Ulcerative Colitis**

At the time of presentation of ulcerative colitis, the disease is limited to the rectum in about 15% of the cases. As the disease progresses, various parts of the colon may be involved, but rectal sparing is fairly uncommon.

301 **Celebrities Are Not Always Heroes**

Help your children understand the differences between heroes and celebrities. Ask them to tell you about their heroes.

302 **Day Care Workers Wash Your Hands**

Day care workers who care for children should touch nothing until they have washed their hands after handling a child with upper respiratory infection, vomiting, or diarrhea.

303 **Different Folks Want Different Information**

Frequently all the patient wants to know is that "this virus is going around." This way they do not feel so isolated. A few patients want you to be more specific: herpes 6 or 7, respiratory syncytial virus, echo, parvo B19, cytomegalovirus, or rotavirus, and so on.

304 **Eventually (Nearly) Everything Passes**

At least 95% of foreign bodies that reach the stomach pass uneventfully. Warn parents that it may take a few weeks to pass larger objects.

305 **Perianal Disease Equals Crohn's Disease**

Perianal disease occurs in Crohn's disease, not in ulcerative colitis.

306 **Chickenpox Pneumonia**

Chickenpox is more likely to cause pneumonia in adults than in children. This disease may cause miliary calcifications on chest x-ray.

307 **Spiral Fractures = Child Abuse**

A child with spiral fracture of a limb has been abused until proved otherwise.

308 **Alternative Therapies on the Rise**

In 1996, more than 40% of Americans used alternative or nonconventional therapies, including herbs, acupuncture, and meditation.

309 **Urinary Tract Infections in Adolescent Girls**

Sexually active adolescent girls have a high incidence of urinary tract infections. About one-third of adolescent girls presenting with dysuria have vaginitis.

310 **Head Injuries and CSF Leakage**

- Clear rhinorrhea after a head injury may or may not be leaking cerebrospinal fluid. Do a dipstick for glucose; if positive, the fluid is CSF.
- If blood clots are in the external ear canal after a head injury, there is probably not a CSF leak into the ear canal.

311 **Teach Vocabulary Whenever You Can**

Teach vocabulary by using some words that young children are not likely to hear elsewhere. For example, use appropriate words to explain why a child's behavior is unacceptable by saying it is rude instead of not nice.

312 **Bag Urine**

Urine specimens collected in plastic bags in the office are useful. The urine specimen should be viewed personally by the doctor if there is any question about the results. Negative test results can be helpful.

313 **Let Parents Look through the Microscope**

If the urine is loaded with white and/or red cells, ask the patient or parents if they would like to look at the microscopic findings themselves. This helps them to understand the problem.

314 **Ask Your Colleagues to Share**

When talking with your fellow pediatricians ask them about the most interesting patient that they have seen in the past few months. You can learn a lot!

315 **UTI in Young Patients**

The younger the patient with a urinary tract infection, the greater the risk of upper tract infection.

316 **Ibuprofen vs. Acetaminophen in Migraine**

In one study of 84 children with migraine, ibuprofen (Advil) was twice as likely as acetaminophen (Tylenol) to abort migraine within 2 hours.

317 **Olive Oil and Cholesterol**

Olive oil may boost good cholesterol and lower bad cholesterol.

318 **Success of Others**

Be generous. Take pleasure in others' success.

319 **Show Patients Their X-rays**

All patients should have the opportunity to view their x-rays and have the problem areas marked. They appreciate the extra time it takes.

320 **Heroes for Children**

Find and tell your children stories about heroes—not superheroes, but real people who do brave things for the common good.

321 **There Is No Place like Home**

Never put a child in the hospital for tests and treatments that can be done at home. In most cases, home and office care is the best.

322 **Drug Costs Vary a Lot**

Never write a prescription until you know what type of insurance (drug card, copayment, full payment) the patient has. For instance, if the patient has chronic allergic rhinitis and you want to prescribe a daily antihistamine, write the prescription for 100 tablets (instead of 30 or 50) if they have a $5 or $10 copayment. The cost of 30 or 50 or 100 may be the same!

323 **Rice vs. Wheat**

A rice-based diet is healthier in children than a diet centered on wheat-based products such as pasta, bread, and cereal.

324 **Nicotine Patches**

Two conditions that may improve with the use of nicotine patches: tics and ulcerative colitis.

325 **Terrific People**

No matter how hard you work to reach your goals, life is not lived to its fullest until it is well sprinkled with terrific people. Terrific people bring out the best in you.

326 **Detail People**

Be nice to drug representatives who visit your office. It is hard to make a living trying to persuade doctors to use your cough and cold medicine. Besides, they can be a good source of referrals.

327 **Meckel's Diverticulum (Rule of Twos)**

Anemia accompanied by hematochezia suggests a Meckel's diverticulum, which according to the *rule of twos*, occurs in 2% of births, is 2 inches (5 cm) long, located 2 feet (60 cm) proximal to the ileocecal valve, and is 2 times more common in males than in females.

328 **CDC Risk Behavior Survey**

The Centers for Disease Control and Prevention is a great source for useful information. Here are some parts of the 1995 Youth Risk Behavior Survey (which sampled over 10,000 adolescents from all over the United States).

1. *Suicide:* 24% of students had seriously considered suicide in the 12 months preceding the survey. Females were at greater risk than males.
2. *Sexual activity:* 53% of students had intercourse at least once, 9% had started before age 13, 18% had sex with 4 or more partners, and 38% had sex within the past 3 months. Fifty-four percent reported using a condom the last time they had sex, and 17% said they or their partners had used oral contraceptives at the time.
3. Substance abuse: 71% of students had tried cigarette smoking at least once; 16% had smoked

CDC Risk Behavior Survey (*Continued*)

cigarettes on 20 or more of the 30 days preceding the survey. Eighteen percent had at least one drink of alcohol in their lifetime, and 33% had five or more drinks on at least one occasion in the 30 days preceding the survey. Forty-two percent had used marijuana during their lifetime, and 25% had used it in the preceding 30 days. For cocaine use, the figures were 7% and 3%. Smaller numbers reported unprescribed steroids use (4%) and illegal injected drug use (2%). Twenty-one percent reported inhalant use, including glue sniffing, breathing from aerosol spray cans, or pain sprays.

4. *Vehicular safety:* 22% of students rarely or never used safety belts when riding in a truck or car driven by someone else. Male students were less likely to use safety belts than females. Among the

CDC Risk Behavior Survey (*Continued*)

25% who had ridden a motorcycle during the preceding year, 44% had rarely or never worn a motorcycle helmet. Of the 76% who rode a bicycle during that time, 93% did not wear bicycle helmets. In the 30 days preceding the survey, 15% had driven a vehicle after drinking alcohol, and 39% had ridden in a vehicle driven by someone who had been drinking, Twenty-two percent reported carrying a weapon to school in the previous 30 days, and 39% had been in a physical fight during that time; both behaviors were much more common among male students.

These findings are reflections of our society. How do you think we are doing? Are medical schools putting enough emphasis on major problems?

329 **Second Most Frequently Prescribed Antimicrobial**

Trimethoprim-sulfamethoxazole (TMP-SMX) is the second most frequently prescribed antimicrobial in the U.S. pediatric population. Rash is its most common adverse effect, occurring in about 1% of treatment courses. (Amoxil is the most common antimicrobial.)

330 **Nonketotic Hypoglycemia**

Currently there are 12 known disorders of mitochondrial beta-oxidation of fatty acids. The hallmark of these disorders is <u>hypoglycemia without urinary ketones in times of fasting or stress</u>.

331 **Hair Growth and Nits**

The egg is laid close to the scalp (at a distance of 1 mm). Hair grows at a rate of 0.40 mm per day. Therefore, any nit more than 6.35 mm from the scalp is not prone to produce a larva and hence is of no clinical significance.

332 **Hypothermia for Brain Trauma?**

There is evidence that hypothermia hastens neurologic recovery in patients with traumatic brain injury.

333 **Kawasaki's Heart Disease Passes Rheumatic Heart Disease**

Kawasaki's disease has now replaced rheumatic fever as the leading cause of acquired heart disease in children in the United States. The most serious complication is development of coronary aneurysms.

334 **Incidence of Down's Syndrome**

The incidence of Down's syndrome in pregnancies steadily rose from 1990 to 1995, increasing from 1.9 per 1000 pregnancies in 1990 to 5.8 per 1000 pregnancies in 1995. It is believed to be attributable to the increasing age of women when they become pregnant.

335 **The Brain Is the Center for Learning**

The cause of learning disabilities lies in the brain, not in the eyeballs. Eye exercises do not help much of anything; they are costly and worthless.

336 **Myths about Teething**

Teething does not cause diarrhea or fever. God would not do that to little babies.

337 **Almost No Eye Problem Causes Learning Disorders**

There is no good evidence that poor vision, jerky eye movements, strabismus, or poor hand–eye coordination causes any learning disabilities.

338 **Foot Care in Athlete's Foot**

Keeping feet dry and avoiding nicks and cuts are essential to successful long-term therapy for athlete's foot.

339 **Congestive Heart Failure in Infants**

Congestive heart failure is identified in infants suspected of heart disease through some combination of findings along a continuum from earliest to latest:

- Difficulty taking formula in infants (i.e., cannot breathe and suck simultaneously, with or without growth failure)
- Tachycardia
- Tachypnea
- Respiratory distress
- Cardiomegaly
- Hepatomegaly
- Rales from pulmonary edema, decreased perfusion, and peripheral edema are late findings in children; their absence should not delay diagnosis.

Dr. John Phillips of Vanderbilt
University School of Medicine

If children live with tolerance,
they learn patience.

From "Children Learn What They Live"

340 **Learning Disorders: Still a Mystery**

The brain of learning-disabled children is "poorly wired" in some unknown way. They have trouble storing and retrieving written information as well as problems decoding words. There is a genetic basis in many cases. Obviously these statements do not apply to cases of acquired learning disabilities following meningitis, head trauma, or drug abuse.

341 **Managed Care**

The most desirable pediatricians for an HMO group are those who "understand realities of managed care" and limit their participation in other plans. The HMOs want doctors who understand "the economic realities of managed care . . . that is a fixed-sum game, in which every dollar spent on hospitalization or ancillary services is not available for physician's fees."

342 **Age of Menarche Correlates with Period of Anovulation**

The later the age of menarche, the longer the period of anovulation.

343 **Tampon Use**

The mean age of tampon use is around 14 years of age. The best predictors of tampon use is favorable maternal attitude and friends' use of tampons.

344 **Anovulatory Cycles**

About 50% of adolescent cycles are anovulatory in the first 2 years after menarche. By 5 years after menarche, about 80% of cycles are ovulatory.

345 **Girl Scout Cookies**

Always buy Girl Scout cookies.

346 **Antibiotics or Not**

In pediatrics about one-third of all prescription drugs are antibiotics. The most important decision in the use of antibiotics is whether they should be used at all.

347 **Myths about Obesity**

The top nutritional problem in kids in the United States is not starvation but obesity. We must dispel the following myths about obesity:

Myth: Obesity is caused by massive overeating. (As little as 100 extra calories per day—6-oz glass of milk—may cause a 10 pound weight gain in 1 year.)

Myth: Obese children eat more junk food and more starch than thin children.

Myth: Obese children overeat because they are upset.

Myth: Obese children store excessive calories in fat, whereas lean children burn calories off.

Myths about Obesity (*Continued*)

Myth: Parents do not care about their child's obesity (They care very much and they are frequently obese themselves.)

Myth: Obesity is not treatable ("I gain it all back and more next year").

The goal of diet, exercise, and other therapies should be good health, not the achievement of an arbitrary set of weights.

348 **Keflex Not for Sinusitis**

Cephalexin (Keflex) does not penetrate sinuses and provides poor *Hemophilus influenzae* coverage.

349 ***Moraxella catarrhalis* in Sinus Infections**

In sinus infections, *Moraxella catarrhalis* is rapidly self-curing and no special prescription has been effective.

350 **Small Children Prone to Hypoglycemia**

Small children have limited glycogen stores and develop hypoglycemia rapidly during periods of stress.

351 **Food Intolerance vs. Food Allergy**

Many patients and some doctors confuse food allergies and food intolerance.

1. Food allergy is caused by type I (IgE-mediated) hypersensitivity. Peanuts are a good example; a person who is allergic to peanuts has a sudden IgE-mediated reaction that may involve the airway with dire consequences.
2. True food allergy is not a common problem. Skin testing is not the best approach to this problem. A negative skin test is a fair predictor that a child does not have a food allergy, but positive results are inconclusive.

Food Intolerance vs. Food Allergy (*Continued*)

3. Many foods are implicated in food allergy but only a few foods cause the majority of reactions. Eggs (especially egg white), soy, wheat, and peanuts cause 85% of food allergies in children. Add shellfish, fish, and tree nuts, and about 95% of food allergies are covered.
4. Children often outgrow allergies to egg, milk, soy, and wheat but not to other foods. A child is much more likely to outgrow an allergy if symptoms start before 3 years of age than if onset comes later.

352 **Dare to Discipline**

Advise all parents to get the book *Dare to Discipline* by James Dobson. When parents, grandparents, and in-laws disagree about spanking and other forms of discipline, this book is helpful.

353 **Know Your Ticks**

Tick paralysis only comes from female tick bites.

354 **Head Lice Second to the Common Cold**

With the exception of the common cold, pediculosis (head lice) affects more school-aged children than all other communicable childhood diseases. Head lice seem to be getting resistant to usual treatments (e.g., Nix, Kwell, permethrin 5% [Elimite]). If you are getting desperate, cover the entire scalp with vaseline and a shower cap for one night. This treatment asphyxiates the mites and the nits.

355 **Supraventricular Tachycardia**

Supraventricular tachycardia is the most common pediatric arrhythmia and is characterized by a rapid fixed heart rate (> 220) and narrow QRS complexes.

356 **Polycystic Kidney Disease**

Autosomal-dominant polycystic kidney disease is the most common inherited renal disease.

357 **Hepatitis C and Chronic Hepatitis**

The most important feature of hepatitis C virus infection is that about 70% of infected patients develop chronic hepatitis.

358 **Repeat Positive Dipsticks**

In an asymptomatic child who tests positive on a random dipstick test for proteinuria, the test should be repeated two or more times before an extensive evaluation is begun. Also consider a split collection with one specimen in the morning on arising and one at bedtime. If the morning specimen is negative and the evening specimen is positive, orthostatic proteinuria is present.

359 **Drug-resistant *S. pneumoniae***

The most consistently identified risk factor for emergence of drug-resistant *Streptococcus pneumoniae* is prior antibiotic use.

360 **CMV: The Most Common Congenital Viral Infection**

Cytomegalovirus (CMV) is the most common congenital infection in infants and children in the United States and is also the most common cause of viral-induced mental retardation and sensorineural deafness.

361 **Carbohydrate Content: Most Common Formula Intolerance**

Although formula intolerance may be related to the carbohydrate, protein, or fat content of milk, by far the most common intolerance is to carbohydrate, specifically lactose.

362 **Good Follow-up**

The pediatrician's best friend is good follow-up.

363 **Digoxin in Wolff-Parkinson-White Syndrome**

Continued use of digoxin therapy in the child over 1 year of age with WPW syndrome is controversial.

364 **Risk of Teenage Pregnancy**

Certain factors increase the risk of teenage pregnancy: poverty, poor intellectual ability, low motivation and expectations, and inadequate schools.

365 **Lead Poisoning from Paint**

Lead-based paint is the predominant source of lead, and paint chips and lead-contaminated house dust are the primary vectors of lead poisoning.

366 **Long QT Syndrome**

Patients who present with syncope and seizures should have a full electrocardiographic study to screen for congenital long QT syndrome.

367 **Eyes Open or Closed?**

- Patients with nonspecific abdominal pain often keep their eyes closed during palpation of the abdomen.
- Patients with organic illnesses usually keep their eyes open.

368 **Enuresis: Workup or Not?**

Children younger than 7 years with enuresis, who have a normal history, physical examination, and urinalysis, do not require further evaluation. The family and patient need reassurance about the enuresis. Always ask if the child can pass a good stream (no dribbling).

369 **Family Photographs in Your Office**

Keep a photo of your children and spouse visible at work if at all possible. When family members come to visit, they will quickly see that they are not forgotten and that you want to show them off.

370 **Use Inhaled Corticosteroids Regularly**

Inhaled corticosteroids are mainly effective when used regularly. They do not provide immediate relief of symptoms. Albuterol is better for acute attacks; steroids are best for their antiinflammatory properties.

371 **Herpes Simplex and Erythema Multiforme**

The typical course of herpes simplex virus-associated erythema multiforme in childhood is an abrupt onset of more than 100 red papules, with most of the lesions on the upper extremities.

372 **Activated Charcoal vs. Gastric Evacuation**

In recent years, the trend in gastric decontamination has been away from gastric evacuation and toward the use of activated charcoal alone.

373 **Perinatally Acquired AIDS**

The number of reported cases of perinatally acquired (mother-to-infant) AIDS declined by 27% between 1992 and 1995 (CDC data). Increased use of perinatal zidovudine (AZT) by HIV-infected pregnant women and their newborns is the most likely factor leading to this reduction.

374 **Scabies and Pruritus**

The main symptom of scabies is pruritus, which is not directly caused by the burrowing mites or larva but by the allergic reaction of hosts once they become sensitized.

375 **Enuresis Treatment**

After considering cost and possible side effects, the conditioning alarm may be the first choice of treatment for enuresis. Proper education and patience are imperative.

376 **Genes and Body Weight**

Several genes appear to be responsible for the regulation of body weight.

377 **Obesity and Hypertension**

Obesity causes about one-third of all cases of adult hypertension.

378 **Urine Cultures: The Gold Standard for UTI**

It cannot be emphasized enough that the urine culture is the single most reliable means of diagnosing urinary tract infections.

379 **Vascular Malformations vs. Hemangiomas**

The first step in the characterization of vascular birthmarks is to differentiate vascular malformations from hemangiomas.

380 **Cerebral Edema in Diabetic Ketoacidosis**

One of the most devastating complications of diabetic ketoacidosis in the pediatric population is the development of cerebral edema.

381 **More on Familial Mood Disorders**

Depression: when one identical twin has a mood disorder, there is about 50% chance that the other twin will develop the illness at some time. Adopted children whose natural parents had a mood disorder have a three-fold increased incidence of depressive illness compared with the natural children of their adoptive parents.

382 **Obesity: Environment vs. Heredity**

Eighty percent of children born to two obese parents will become obese compared with 14% of children born to normal-weight parents. Studies comparing the weight of adoptees to the weights of biologic and adopted parents indicate that genetic factors are responsible for only 33% of the variance in weight.

383 **Congenital Glaucoma**

Tearing, sensitivity to light, corneal clouding, and progressive enlargement of the eye are the main clinical manifestations of congenital glaucoma.

384 **Alport's Syndrome of Nephritis and Deafness**

Alport's syndrome (hereditary nephritis and deafness) has an X-linked dominant pattern of inheritance; males are more severely affected than females.

385 **Teenage Pregnancy**

About 70% of teenage girls' babies are fathered by men at least 5 years older than the girl.

386 **Progenitor of End-Stage Renal Disease**

Posterior urethral valves represent the most important renal disorder detectable in early childhood with regard to potential for progression to end-stage renal disease.

387 **Small Cuts**

Parents need not rush off to the emergency department for every small laceration. Pinch the edges of the cut together. When the bleeding has stopped, take clear scotch tape and put it across the wound (perpendicular to the cut). This technique works much better than butterflies, which most parents do not have at their disposal anyway.

388 **Pediatric Journals**

Pediatric Annals and *Contemporary Pediatrics* have very helpful articles for doctors in practice.

389 **Some Facts about Diets**

- A high-carbohydrate, low-fat diet is most effective for weight loss.
- Low-fat diets contain more food for the same number of calories than high-fat diets.
- In one major study, calorie for calorie, the most satisfying foods were high in fiber. Potatoes were the most satisfying of the 17 foods tested.

390 **Depression and Anxiety: Common**

Depression and anxiety disorders are common. Ten percent of Americans experience a significant mood disorder (usually depression) at some time in their life.

391 **New Teaching Device for Teenagers**

Have teenagers pull a token from a sack that is passed to each member of the class. The tokens represent the incidence of HIV, gonococcus, and other sexually transmitted diseases in the area and the risk of pregnancy. One token may say "You're lucky this time," another may say "HIV" or "pregnancy." As the sack progresses around the room, students get a realistic picture of just how risky sex is—protected or not, even the first time. Pass the sack around a few more times and the impact grows.

392 **Rotavirus Diarrhea**

Rotavirus infection is estimated to cause about 3 million cases of diarrhea yearly; about 64,000 of patients are hospitalized. About 125 deaths annually in the United States are due to rotavirus.

393 **Maternal Drugs in Meconium**

Meconium can be used to detect cocaine, marijuana, opiates, and a score of other drugs. These drugs stay in meconium even though they were not used by the mother within the past 20 weeks before delivery of a term infant.

394 **Panic Attacks**

- The prevalence of panic disorder is 1–2% in both men and women. These attacks begin in the late teens or early 20s. One estimate suggests that only 25% of people with panic attacks receive appropriate care.
- The cardinal features of panic disorder are short-lived, sudden, unexpected attacks of terror and fear of losing control; attacks begin without warning during non-threatening activities.
- An attack generally peaks within 10 minutes and dissipates within 20 to 30 minutes.

395 **Galactosemia: Not as Treatable as We Thought**

The early diagnosis of galactosemia and the use of a galactose-restricted diet have not had the expected long-term success. A group in London reported that 50% of patients over 6 years of age were developmentally delayed and that learning difficulties increased with age. Eighty percent of the females also had gonadal failure.

396 **Poverty and Teenage Pregnancy**

Forty percent of U.S. girls live near or below poverty income levels and account for 80% of out-of-wedlock births.

397 **Oxygen Use in Respiratory Emergencies**

All respiratory emergency patients should receive 100% oxygen until the initial assessment of respiratory function is made.

398 **Smell: Most Primitive Sense**

Smell is the most primitive of the senses. It has no cortical representation; instead, the reception and interpretation of odors are confined to the limbic system.

399 **Chorioamnionitis in Preterm Infants**

Chorioamnionitis is present in preterm delivery in up to 50% of infants with very low birth weight.

400 **Salmeterol (Long-acting) Inhaler**

Salmeterol (Serevent) is a good inhaler to use at night for asthma because it lasts all night (albuterol lasts only about 3–4 hours).

401 **Vesicoureteral Reflux**

Vesicoureteral reflux that persists when inflammation resolves (4–6 weeks) is often familial.

402 **Infertility in Males**

Infertility effects 1 man in 25. In about 30–40% of affected men, the results of semen analysis are abnormal, but no cause of the infertility can be found.

403 **Ehrlichiosis**

The first case of ehrlichiosis in the United States was reported in 1986. This acute febrile illness follows a tick bite. Unlike Lyme disease, however, it is usually accompanied by leukopenia, thrombocytopenia, and elevated serum aminotransferase level.

404 **Leave the Child in the Bed**

If a child is crying at 2 A.M. but is not sick, pat and reassure the child but do not get the child out of bed. That can start a bad cycle. Do not let the child sleep in your bed; then no one sleeps.

405 **HIV in Children**

As recently as 1996, a total of approximately 20,000 children in the United States and 1.5 million children worldwide were infected with HIV.

406 **Structural Brain Changes in Anorexia**

Brain-imaging studies have shown evidence of ventricular and sulcal enlargement in patients with anorexia nervosa. Similar changes have been noted in patients on long-term or high-dose corticosteroids.

407 **Teenage Suicides and Murders**

American teenagers are now killing themselves (suicide) and other teenagers (murder) more frequently than teenagers in any other industrial country in the world. Why? Is it related to television or movies? Write us if you know the answer.

408 **Memory Impairment in Brain Injury**

Memory impairment is the most common cognitive deficit after brain injury in children.

409 **Chlamydial Pneumonia**

Chlamydial pneumonia usually occurs after 3 weeks of age and is accompanied by or recently associated with conjunctivitis in up to 50% of cases. Chlamydial pneumonia has an insidious onset. Infants present with tachypnea and prominent cough but are almost always afebrile. Chest exam reveals rales and a few wheezes. A frequently associated and distinctive laboratory finding is eosinophilia (greater than 400 cells/mm).

410 **Group A Streptococci: Not from Dogs or Cats**

The family pet is an unlikely source of group A streptococcal infections in humans.

411 **Siblings of Infants with FUO**

When you have a small baby with fever of unknown origin, ask the mother what problems the siblings have had in the last 5–10 days. The answer is usually a great help.

412 **Age at Menarche**

The average girl starts menses at 12.8 years. She generally starts ovulation about 2 years later. Clinically she may note bloating and discomfort at the time of ovulation.

413 **Thrush Treatment**

If you cannot clear a baby's oral thrush with nystatin, try fluconazole (Diflucan). Gentian violet is still good treatment but messy.

414 **Alcohol Swabs May Be Outdated**

Recent evidence shows that routine use of alcohol swabs before injections and venipuncture is of little value. Use Betadine.

415 **Treat What Hurts**

Always treat the chief complaint. For example, do not treat otitis with antibiotics alone. Give something for the pain.

416 **Store Medicines in Safe Place**

Iron supplements are the most common cause of poisoning deaths in children.

417 **Gaucher's Disease**

Gaucher's disease (most common in Ashkenazi Jews) is the most common lysosomal storage disorder.

418 **Hug Children**

Show your children affection. Hugging, kissing, and cuddling your children show that they are important and mean a lot to you.

419 **Be Gentle**

Never approach a child with an otoscope. First put the scope in the parent's ear so that the child can see that it does not hurt.

420 **Likewise with the Stethoscope**

First put the stethoscope on the parent's chest.

421 **Meconium Peritonitis**

The ability of ultrasound to pick up calcification is the principal reason that we can now diagnose meconium peritonitis *in utero*.

422 **Bathing Young Children**
Never leave a young child alone in the bath.

423 **Pay for What Doctors Do *for* Patients**
Doctors need to be paid for what they do *for* patients, rather than what they do *to* patients.

424 **Safety around the House**
If you must keep a gun in the house (which should be avoided whenever possible), keep it unloaded and locked up. Lock ammunition in a separate location.

425 **Guns and Teenagers**
American teenagers are 12 times more likely to die from a gun than teenagers from other industrial countries. Why? Is it related to television or movies? Write us if you know the answer.

426 **Specialize in Something**

As you go about your daily practice, try to find one area in which, with extra study and work, you can be among the best. Pick an area that fascinates you.

427 **Immunoglobulins in Infants**

IgG is the only class of immunoglobulin transferred across the placenta. Infants can synthesize IgA and IgM. Premature infants are significantly hypogammaglobulinemic (low IgG).

428 **Guillain-Barré Syndrome**

Various causes of Guillain-Barré syndrome have been implicated. It has been associated with *Campylobacter* infections, cerebrovascular accidents, cytomegalovirus infections, and insect stings. It has been associated with swine-influenza vaccine but not the measles vaccine.

429 **Good First-line Treatment for Urinary Tract Infections**

Trimethoprim-sulfamethoxazole is a good first-line drug for urinary tract infections (usually *Escherichia coli* infections in children).

430 **Malignancy: Not a Common Cause of FUO in Children**

Malignancy is a less likely cause of fever of unknown origin in children than in adults.

431 **Do Not Drive and Talk on Telephones**

About one vehicle collision every 10 minutes in the United States results in a fatality. An error on the part of drivers contributes to over 90% of these events. A significant number of the involved drivers were using cellular telephones at the time of or just before the accident.

432 **Hemorrhagic Cystitis**

Adenovirus (type II) is a cause of hemorrhagic cystitis in children.

433 **Potty Chair Wisdom**

Whenever a child is sitting on a potty chair against his or her will, we are all wasting our time.

434 **Apnea**

Apnea is the cessation of respiration for 10–20 seconds with or without bradycardia or cyanosis. Any color change or spells lasting longer than 15–20 seconds signify critical illness.

435 **More about Lyme Disease**

Lyme disease is the most common vector-borne disease in the United States.

436 **Sedimentation Rate in Kawasaki Disease**

If the sedimentation rate is less than 40 mm/hour, you probably are not dealing with Kawasaki's disease.

437 **Glasses Do Not Fix Everything**

Neither eye exercises nor glasses will cure a child who reverses letters.

438 **Sit with Patients**

On hospital rounds, sit on the patient's bed. Even if you are rushed, your haste will not be apparent.

439 **Time Moves Slowly in ADHD**

Children with attention deficit hyperactivity disorder seem to perceive time as moving more slowly than it actually does. They are going to arrive late for nearly every event. They usually are not punctual and do not meet deadlines. They are impatient for the same reasons.

440 **Commit to Community Service**

Find a need in your community and commit yourself to it. Strive toward that goal. Dr. Bob Sanders (a local pediatrician) made Tennessee the first state in the United States to require safety seat belts for children.

441 **No Hot Tubs in Pregnancy**

Avoid hot tubs and saunas during the first 6 months of pregnancy.

442 **Use Language Therapeutically**

- "Those headaches you *had*, what did you do to make them go away?"
- "What part of the stomachache will you want to *change* first?"
- "Would it be okay *if the hurt did not bother you?*"
- "So when you keep the bed dry, *what do you do?*"

443 **Pansinusitis in Cystic Fibrosis**

Pansinusitis is almost universal in cystic fibrosis.

444 **Aspermia and Cystic Fibrosis**

Obstructive azoospermia constitutes strong evidence for cystic fibrosis.

445 **Ultrasound in FUO**

If your evaluation of a patient with fever of unknown origin has not been productive in the first 2 days, consider ultrasonography of the abdomen and possibly computerized tomography of the abdomen. If these tests are normal, repeat the entire history again.

446 **If You Want Your Child to Attend Religious Services**

If you do not attend, your children probably will not attend. Parents teach best by example.

447 **Tinea Capitis Increasing**

Cases of tinea capitis are increasing around the country, especially among children in the inner cities. Griseofulvin is the first line of treatment. Topical treatment alone is not effective.

448 **BB Guns Are Not Toys**

Many BB guns can propel pellets at the same speeds at which conventional gunpowder firearms discharge their ammunition. BB guns are not toys.

449 **More about Guns**

A study at Northwestern University showed that one family in five had a handgun in the house. One in ten of these families leaves the gun lying around loaded. Fifteen hundred people are killed each year by unintentional firearm discharge injuries.

450 **Friends**

Real friends are made one at a time, usually through shared activity.

451 **Now Hear This**

- There are 24.5 million visits per year for otitis media.
- Antibiotic costs alone are $240 million.
- Many doctors (especially the British) say we are treating a disease in which 25% or more of cases spontaneously improve.

452 **Endocardial Fibroelastosis and Mumps**

Endocardial fibroelastosis (EFE) was a common form of heart disease until about 1980 but has declined dramatically. The reason may be linked to the mumps vaccine introduced in 1968. The mumps virus appears to have caused most cases of EFE.

453 **Adenoviruses and myocarditis**

Adenoviruses are now the most common causes of viral myocarditis in children. Coxsackie viruses are the second most common cause.

454 **Spanking Decreasing**

In the last decade, the number of parents using spanking as a way of discipline is decreasing. The alternative to spanking, time out, has gained popularity over the past several years.

455 **Asthma Increasing**

The leading chronic illness among American children is asthma. It affects about 4.8 million youngsters under the age of 18. The number of cases has risen nearly 80% in the last 15 years, according to the American Lung Association. The reasons are not entirely clear.

456 **Vocabulary Development**

Babies understand more than they can say at first. Do not be discouraged if your child's first words take time. Speak to your child as much as possible. During the second year, the child discovers that everything has a name. The vocabulary grows rapidly.

Age:	*Average number of words:*
12 months	3
18 months	22
2 years	272
3 years	896

457 **A Sign of Allergy**

A child who comes to the office with a sack full of drugs is an allergic child until proved otherwise. A child with ear tubes before one year of age is usually an allergic child.

458 **Drug Toxicity**

A recent study showed that adverse drug events cost more than $100 billion per year and account for 140,000 deaths annually.

459 **Don't Be Vague**

Eliminate vague instructions such as "use as directed."

460 **Caddies and Lyme Disease**

In endemic areas, caddies of high-handicap golfers are more prone to tick bites and thus to Lyme disease. They spend more time in the rough and woods.

461 **Calories Count**

Low-fat food can make you fat if you eat too much of it. A calorie is a calorie, whether it comes from fat, protein, or carbohydrates.

462 **Women Live Longer than Men**

Seventy-five percent of women outlive their husbands.

463 **Read to Children**

The more often you read aloud—and the more advanced the books are—the easier it becomes for your child to understand complex ideas.

464 **More about Otitis Media**

Otitis media accounts for more visits to pediatricians than any other illness (24.4 million in 1990, up almost 150% since 1975).

465 **Navel Pointers**

In children with abdominal pain, the closer they point with one finger to their navel, the less likely they are to have a disease that can be demonstrated.

466 **Grandparents**

It takes a whole village to replace a single grandparent.

467 **Television for Toddlers**

By age two, American kids spend an average of 27 hours per week in front of the television. Television viewing is used too much as a baby sitter.

468 **Good Day Care Hard to Find**

Thirty percent of all parents say that finding good day care has been a problem. Thirty percent say that they have had trouble finding a job with flexible time options.

469 **Parents and Sunday School**

Eighty percent of all mothers and 74% of all fathers say that they plan to send their child to Sunday School or some other kind of religious training.

470 **Pediatricians: Limit Television**

The American Academy of Pediatrics advises parents to limit television time to 1–2 hours a day (with careful choice of what they watch).

471 **Breath-holder? Try Iron Treatment**

Iron deficiency anemia may lead to adverse effects on brain tissue. Several studies have found that a fair number of children with breath-holding spells are iron-deficient. <u>Iron therapy reduces the number and intensity of breath-holding spells</u>.

472 **Petit Mal**

If you think a child has petit mal, ask the child to hyperventilate for a while. If the child develops a blank "stare attack," you do not need an electroencephalogram to make the diagnosis. You just made it.

473 **_H. pylori_ in Endoscoped Children**

Studies in pediatric populations have determined that 15% of all children undergoing endoscopy and gastric biopsy have evidence of *Helicobacter pylori* infection.

474 **Some Facts about Cytomegalovirus**

- CMV is the leading cause of congenital viral infections in the United States.
- CMV involves 1% of all newborns (or about 40,000 babies per year).
- About 90–95% of infected babies have no evidence of disease in the newborn period.
- Sensorineural hearing loss is the most common complication. About 4,000 children acquire hearing loss every year from CMV infections.
- In a few, deterioration of hearing continues even after 6 years of age. Amazing!

475 **Where Can Parents Get Outside Help?**
(*Newsweek*, Special Issue, Spring 1997)

On the Phone:

- **Child Care Aware**
  800-424-2246
  Operators refer parents anywhere in the country to licensed and accredited childcare centers in their area.
- **ChildHelp National Hotline**
  800-4-A-CHILD
  Twenty-four-hour advice and referrals for children and adults with questions or in crisis.
- **Gerber Information Line**
  800-443-7237
  Tipper Gore's recorded welcome message jolts you from thoughts of strained peas on this 24-hour consumer-info line.

Where Can Parents Get Outside Help? (*Continued*)

- **National Parent Information Network**
  800-583-4135
  NPIN boasts the largest parenting database in the country. Researchers hunt down referrals, abstracts, and answers and send them free of charge to hundreds of callers every month.
- **Parents Anonymous**
  909-621-6184 (not toll-free)
  The national office in Claremont, California, refers parents to 45 state and regional affiliates, which offer support groups, counseling, and referrals.
- **Single Parents Association**
  800-704-2102
  This line, which has just gone national, helps parents find support groups and resources in their communities.

Where Can Parents Get Outside Help? (*Continued*)

On the Internet:

- **Usenet**
  alt.parenting and misc.kids
  Great places to start on the usenet—the Internet's collection of newsgroups; discussions on hundreds of topics.
- **Childbirth.Org**
  http://www.childbirth.org
  Top discussion forums and a home page that get right to the point on tough issues.
- **Family.com**
  http://www.family.com
  Disney's new site has been criticized for being more upscale than helpful.

Where Can Parents Get Outside Help? (*Continued*)

- **ParenTalk Newsletter**
  http://www.tnpc.com/parentalk/index.html
  Clearly written articles by physicians and psychologists. What this site lacks in graphic creativity, it makes up for in sheer mass of information.
- **ParenthoodWeb**
  http://parenthoodweb.com
  Pediatricians and psychiatrists respond (in due time) to your e-mail.
- **Parenting Q&A**
  http://www.parenting-qa.com
  This site calls itself the only one on the Web "solely devoted to providing parents with answers to their most pressing questions."

Where Can Parents Get Outside Help? (*Continued*)

- **ParentSoup**
  http://www.parentsoup.com
  Excellent discussion forums.
- **Zero to Three**
  http://www.zerotothree.org
  The Washington, D.C.-based child advocacy group has just launched its web site. A wealth of research and information about physical, cognitive, and social development of infants and toddlers.

476 **The Whole World Toilet Trains before Us**

Half of the children in the world are toilet-trained by one year of age (but not in the United States), according to Dr. Barton D. Schmitt. Eighteen months is a reasonable time to start toilet training; however, there is no single correct age.

477 **Uveitis in Juvenile Rheumatoid Arthritis**

There seems to be no relationship between the time of appearance of uveitis and the severity of juvenile rheumatoid arthritis. Uveitis may precede the arthritis or appear late in the disease.

478 **Toe Walking May Not Be a Benign Condition**

- Children with autism are frequently toe walkers.
- If a child is a toe walker, look carefully for language delay.
- The presence or history of toe-walking should strongly incline the clinician toward a neurologically based developmental language disorder.

479 **Nurses for Telephone Coverage**

Recent studies have shown that one registered nurse can do after-hours phone coverage for about 15 pediatricians.

480 **Disposable Diapers**

Disposable diapers are probably the leading factor in the trend toward delayed toilet training in the United States.

481 **Babies Use a Lot of Diapers**

The average child consumes about 5,000 diapers before full training.

482 **Milk Protein and Soy Protein Sensitivity**

It is estimated that as many as one-third of milk protein-sensitive infants are also sensitive to soy protein.

483 **Chlamydia on the Rise**

In 1995 almost one-half of chlamydial infections in women occurred among adolescents and one-third occurred among 20–24 year olds (CDC data). The rate of chlamydial infections continues to rise.

484 **Meconium Ileus and Cystic Fibrosis**

The earliest intestinal manifestation of cystic fibrosis is meconium ileus, which may occur in 10–15% of affected infants. It is virtually pathognomonic of cystic fibrosis.

485 **Dipsticks: Not for Diabetic Urines**

Dipsticks to test for protein in urine are not sensitive enough to pick up the early microalbuminuria of diabetic nephropathy.

486 **Strong Odor? Look in the Nose**

Any child with a "strong body odor" has a foreign body in the nose until proved otherwise.

487 **Pacifiers Stop Breast-feeding Early**

Babies who use the pacifier a great deal are likely to stop breast-feeding earlier than nonusers.

488 **Reduce Inflammation in Asthma**

The goal in asthma therapy is to reduce and eliminate chronic bronchial inflammation. This is now done mainly with inhaled steroids, cromolyn, and accolate (Zafirlukast).

489 **Green Hair**

Green hair is caused by uptake of copper by the hair shaft. Prevention: Wash the hair immediately after swimming and maintain the pH of pool water between 7.4 and 7.6.

490 **Self-esteem and Parents**

One source of self-esteem is internal—the young child's own pleasure at having accomplished a task. Another is external—feedback from parents who recognize the child's achievement.

491 **Self-injury in Autism**

Self-injury is a primary reason for institutionalization of people with mental retardation and autism.

492 **Congenital Lactase Deficiency**

Congenital lactase deficiency should be suspected in neonates with congenital diarrhea, poor weight gain, and acidic stools containing reducing sugars.

493 ***Newsweek* (Special Edition, Spring 1997)**

- What is the most important goal for your child? Parents (48%) said, "Making sure he/she grows up to be a moral person."
- What do you worry about most in your child's future? Parents (54%) said, "That he/she will be kidnapped or a victim of a violent crime."

494 **Stool Precautions**
Avoid projectile stools.

495 **Intensive Ballet Training**
Look for the following medical conditions in young girls involved in intensive ballet dance training:

- Decreased growth velocity
- Eating disorders
- Delayed puberty

496 **Raising Prodigies**
If parents want to raise a prodigy, the best they can do is make experiences available to the child.

497 **Learning about Words and Sounds**
Children attach meanings to sounds before they shed their diapers. They analyze grammar by age 3.

498 **Reading, Singing, and Playing Music**

Fifty percent of parents say that they read to their child each day; about the same number say that they sing or play music for their child daily. More parents should do so.

499 **Some Standard Books about Baby Care**

1. *Baby and Child Care* (Dr. Benjamin Spock), Pocket Books, $18.00
2. *What to Expect the First Year—What to Expect the Toddler Years* (Arlene Eisenberg, Heidi Murkoff, Sandee Hathaway), Workman Publishing, $12.95
3. *Your Baby and Child* (Penelope Leach), Knopf, $19.95. Explains things from the baby's point of view. Fun to read.
4. *Touchpoints* (T. Berry Brazelton), Addison Wesley, $14.95. Dr. Brazelton is a model for all pediatricians.

500 **School by Age Three?**

Thirty-three percent of all parents say that they plan to start sending their child to school by the age of three; an additional 30% say that their child will start by age four. (Home schooling at this young age by a parent may be the preferred method.)

501 **Early Computers**

One-fourth of all parents of children 2–3 years old say that their child plays with a computer or computer game three or more times a week.

502 **Giardiasis in Swimming Pools**

Two million people contact giardiasis every year (CDC). Swimming pool outbreaks are common, since *Giardia* species is resistant to chlorine. On a camping trip, boiling water for 12 minute is adequate.

503 **Breast-feeding and IQ**

A series of studies have shown there is a "small increase" (up to an 8 point difference) in IQ in breast-fed babies compared with bottle-fed babies.

504 **Languages and Sounds**

Each of the world's approximately 6,000 languages uses a different assortment of distinctive sounds to build words.

505 **Words Linked to Meanings**

By their first birthday, most children start linking words to meanings.

506 **Stretching in Children?**

Stretching exercises for children before an athletic event is questionable. There are no adequate studies to prove their value. No need to "push them."

507 **Mono: Often Subclinical**

Many cases of mononucleosis due to Epstein-Barr virus (EBV) are subclinical. Most adults in the United States show evidence of previous infection with EBV by serology.

508 **Pain and Early Cancer**

Early cancer is rarely painful.

509 **Pubic Lice in Infants Live on Eyelashes**

Pubic lice live on pubic hair. In infants, infestation is confined to the eyelashes and occasionally scalp hair.

510 **Lessons for the Summertime**

Teach your children not to abandon ship. If your boat gets swamped, stay with it. Boats usually stay afloat and drift to shore. Most people cannot swim as far as they think they can.

511 **Cancer Is Not One Disease**

Cancer is actually a group of about 100 diseases. Each can be caused by many different factors.

512 **Pull-on-the-ear Test**

Pulling on the ear lobe is painful in external otitis (swimmer's ear) but not in otitis media. This test is useful during swimming months, especially when the doctor is called on the phone by a parent.

513 **Liver Makes Most of the Cholesterol**

The liver makes about 80% of the cholesterol in the body. You take in the rest when you eat animal products.

514 **Soybeans: A Cheap Protein**

Soybeans are an inexpensive way to add protein to your diet. Soybeans may also lower cholesterol.

515 **Plasma Cell Granuloma—Most Common Childhood Lung Tumor**

Plasma cell granuloma (PCG)—an inflammatory pseudotumor—is the most common benign lung tumor in childhood.

516 **Get Good Associates**

Surround yourself with good associates, as I have: Dr. Bill Doak, Dr. Roland Gray, Dr. J. C. Anderson, and Dr. Margreete Johnston.

517 **Absence of Skin Lesions in Herpes Encephalitis**

Forty percent of children with disseminated herpes-associated encephalitis have no skin lesions. If the child with encephalitis shows neurologic focal signs, think herpes.

518 **Pinworms and Night**

If pinworms cause rectal itching at night, how do they know when it is dark?

519 **Childhood Syncope: Not Usually Cardiovascular**

In only about 1% of pediatric cases is syncope related to a cardiovascular etiology compared with 25% in adults.

520 **Split Liver Transplants**

Of approximately 4,000 liver transplants last year, about 10% could have been split, making an additional 400–500 livers available to children.

521 **Enuresis Runs in Families**

One-third of fathers and one-fifth of mothers have a history of enuresis. If both parents are enuretic, three-fourths of their children will also wet the bed.

522 **Praise Efforts and Accomplishments**

Encourage parents to praise their children's efforts, not just their accomplishments.

523 **Trichomonas Discharge Is Foul**

Vaginal trichomonas discharge is thin, copious, and frothy (infection with *Monilia* species is usually thick). The most characteristic feature of a "trich" discharge is its bad odor.

524 **Travel Medicine Bag**

When you take a trip with small children, be prepared:

- Phenergan suppositories for vomiting
- Cough medicine
- Bandaids
- Cortisone cream
- Benadryl
- Tylenol
- Sunburn lotion and sunscreen

525 **Imipramine for Enuresis**

Imipramine (Tofranil) tablets have about a 50% cure rate in enuresis. However, many children relapse after discontinuing the drug.

526 **Chlamydial Ophthalmia Neonatorum**

Chlamydia is the most common organism causing ophthalmia neonatorum.

527 **Gallops Mean Overload**

A gallop rhythm usually denotes an overloaded cardiovascular system.

528 **Depression: A Common Disorder**

According to the American Academy of Child and Adolescent Psychiatry, about 5% of children and adolescents have significant depression.

529 **Malingering Pursues a Goal**

Malingering may be defined as symptoms under voluntary control but feigned in pursuit of a goal.

530 **Topical Nasal Steroids**

Use topical nasal steroids in older children with allergic rhinitis. They work well with few side effects. Someone should make a nasal spray with cortisone and cromolyn combined. Watch for the new antihistamine nasal spray, Astelin (azelastine HCl).

531 **No FDA-approved Drugs for Depression under Age 19 Years**

Currently (1997) no medications to treat depression are approved by the Food and Drug Administration for children. However, many of the drugs for adult depression are helpful with depressed children.

532 **Listen for Pneumonia**

Be sure when you listen to the chest of a child with fever and bronchitis to let the parents know that you do not "hear any pneumonia." Pneumonia is what they are worried about. They need to hear that you have listened for it.

533 **Smoking Discouraged in African-American Families**

A Memphis study (7,000 teenagers) showed:

- The age at which white teenagers typically started smoking was the 8th grade.
- African-American children generally did not start experimenting with tobacco until the 10th grade.
- By the 12th grade 30% of children were regular smokers.
- Smoking was discouraged more strongly in African-American families.

534 **Viral Pneumonia**

Most pneumonia in children under two years of age is viral.

535 **Tender TMJ Joints**

Headaches due to a temporomandibular joint (TMJ) disorder are usually associated with tenderness to palpation over the TMJ. Look for other causes of headache if this tenderness is not present.

536 **Mandated Screenings**

- Currently only Rhode Island and Hawaii require all newborns to be screened for deafness before discharge.
- Another 15 states mandate screening only for infants in the intensive care unit.
- Eleven states incorporate newborn screening for congenital adrenal hyperplasia.

537 **Lithium and Alcohol**

Lithium is not effective if the adolescent is drinking alcohol.

538 **Obsessive Compulsive Disorders Are Not Admitted**

About 1 million children have obsessive compulsive disorder. Here is yet another condition not discussed on ward rounds in the past.

539 **Allergy Testing: A Test, Not a Diagnosis**

Allergy testing does not make a diagnosis; it only reveals whether the patient has IgE antibodies to environmental allergens.

540 **Sensitivity to Peanuts Is Long-lasting**

Milk sensitivities are commonly outgrown, but peanut sensitivity lasts for many years.

541 **Antidepressant Prescriptions**

According to the research firm IMS America Ltd., in 1996 about 581,000 children and adolescents received a prescription for fluoxetine (Prozac), paroxetine (Paxil), or sertraline (Zoloft).

542 **Ipecac: The Tried and True Emetic**

Although many agents have been used to induce vomiting, including dilute detergent, hydrogen peroxide, and salt water, syrup of ipecac is the only approved emetic in current use.

543 **Migraine Headaches: Familial**

Migraine is an autosomal dominant trait; therefore, a careful family history is imperative. If patients use the words "sick headache, terrible headaches, throbbing and pounding," they are usually describing migraine.

544 **Deafness and Pneumococcal Meningitis**

About 25% of patients with pneumococcal meningitis develop hearing loss, no matter how early the treatment for meningitis starts.

545 **Alcohol and Hypoglycemia**

A child with unexplained drowsiness, low blood sugar, and a low body temperature may be drunk. Most children do not have a breath odor of alcohol.

546 **Plantar Fasciitis**

Consider using off-the-shelf silicone or rubber heel pads for the heel pain of plantar fasciitis.

547 **Perthes Disease of the Hip**

Ninety percent of patients with Perthes disease of the hip present between 4 and 9 years of age.

548 **Small Doses of Lomotil Can Be Fatal**

As few as 5 Lomotil (diphenoxylate 2.5 mg, atropine 0.025 mg) tablets may cause death in a child. One or two tablets may be fatal in 1–2-year-old children.

549 **Hashimoto's Thyroiditis**

Hashimoto's thyroiditis is the most common cause of goiters in children.

550 **Serum Ferritin**

Serum ferritin is increased in anemia of chronic disease but decreased in iron deficiency anemia.

551 **Mitral Valve Prolapse**

Diastolic clicks are frequently heard with mitral valve prolapse; they may be heard best when the patient is standing.

552 **Hemiplegic Migraine**

Aspirin may relieve hemiplegic migraine. Try it.

553 **Diastolic Murmurs**

All diastolic murmurs are pathologic.

554 **Disappearance of Strawberry Hemangiomas**

Easy way to remember the disappearance of strawberry hemangiomas:

- 50% disappear by age 5
- 70% disappear by age 7
- 90% disappear by age 9

555 **Thyroid Dysgenesis Causes Congenital Hypothyroidism**

Thyroid dysgenesis (ectopic or total agenesis) accounts for about 80% of congenital hypothyroidism in newborns.

If children live with acceptance,
they learn to love.

From "Children Learn What They Live"

556 **Otitis Media and *H. influenzae***

Most *Hemophilus influenzae* organisms causing otitis media are nontypable.

557 **Asthma and Infections**

Exacerbations of asthma tend to be associated with viral, not bacterial infections. However, if an asthmatic patient does not respond to medication, think of an associated bacterial infection, especially sinusitis.

558 **Prescription Mistakes Are Common**

Mistakes on prescriptions are made about 17 million times per year.

559 **Poverty Alone Not Enough**

Poverty alone is not sufficient justification for separating children from their families.

560 **Television Time Adds Up**

By the time today's child reaches age 70, he or she will have spent 7 years watching TV.

561 **Three Major Areas of ADHD**

Attention deficit hyperactivity disorder (ADHD) is divided into 3 major subtypes:

1. Inattention
2. Impulsivity
3. Hyperactivity

562 **School Phobia**

School phobia affects 5% of elementary school students.

563 **Giving to Others**

People who give to others are happier and healthier people. Learn this early and teach it to your children.

564 **Sinks Are Not for Pets**

Do not clean the cages of pets in the kitchen sink.

565 **Ritalin Usage Changing**

Important changes in the last few years in the use of Ritalin (methylphenidate):

- It is <u>used longer</u> now than before—more patients are teenagers and college students.
- It is being <u>used earlier</u> in life, i.e., 4–5 years of age. Ten years ago Ritalin was rarely started until school age.
- Five years ago Ritalin was rarely used more than twice daily; now the day goes better for the entire family if Ritalin is <u>used 3 times</u>/day in many children.
- About 80% of parents believe that their children's school grades benefitted from Ritalin usage.
- There has been a 2–3-fold increase in the number of prescriptions for Ritalin used during 1990–1995.

566 **Pets Lower Blood Pressure**

Studies have shown that people who own pets have lower blood pressure than people who do not. Dog owners have usually fared best, probably because they walked the most.

567 **Earlier Puberty**

A national study of American girls (aged 3–12 years) showed that 48% of African-American girls and nearly 15% of white girls showed signs of puberty (breasts and pubic hair) by age 8.

568 **Asthma: Most Common Chronic Disease in Children**

Asthma is now the most common chronic disease, affecting between 10–15% of children and up to 10% of adults. The incidence is still increasing.

569 **Young Patients with Hypertension**
The younger the patient with hypertension, the more likely a secondary (and often curable) cause can be found (renal disease, coarctation of aorta, and so on).

570 **Smokers Pay for Antismoking Ads**
Three states (Arizona, California, and Massachusetts) presently use money made from an added tax on cigarette sales to promote antismoking campaigns.

571 **Smoking and Car Accidents**
Smokers have twice as many car accidents as nonsmokers.

572 **Most Smokers Start Early**
Eighty percent of all smokers start the habit before 18 years of age. This is a major pediatric disease.

573 **Medical School Curriculum Needs to Get Current**

These following subjects were not commonly taught in the past:

- Attention deficit disorders
- Otitis media
- Asthma
- School failure
- Drug problems (alcohol, marijuana, and tobacco use)
- High school dropouts
- Marriage counseling
- Obesity

The curriculum of medical schools needs to be changed to address these major problems.

574 **Lie Detecting**

The secret of detecting lies is to <u>focus on *how* something is told to you</u> rather than on *what* is said.

575 **Tuberculin Skin Test after Foreign Travel**

All travelers to virtually any country outside the United States should have a tuberculosis skin test on return.

576 **Duration of Drugs in Urine after Ingestion**

- Cocaine: 96–144 hours
- Marijuana: 120 hours from single dose
  240 hours from daily use.

577 **Scabies in Infants**

Elimite (permethrin) cream 5% is indicated for scabies in infants as young as 2 months of age. Apply the cream to the whole body and the hands. If the child is a hand sucker, application should be delayed until the child is asleep.

578 **Pills Do Not Create Skills**

Even when an antidepressant works, it must be accompanied by counseling. Pills do not take away insecurities or create self-esteem.

579 **Pubic Lice and Sexually Transmitted Disease**

About one-third of patients with pubic lice have other sexually transmitted disease.

580 **Drugs for Tics**

Resperidone (Risperdal) may be the drug of choice in some severe tic disorders (Tourette's syndrome, for instance).

581 **Airway Resistance in the Nose**

About 50% of airway resistance from the nostrils to the alveoli occurs in the nose, not the lower airways. Most asthmatics open their mouth to breathe.

582 **Avoid Surgery for Strawberry Hemangiomas**

Less than 2% of strawberry hemangiomas need surgery. Avoid radical treatment unless there is an alarming spurt of growth of the hemangioma.

583 **Immunotherapy**

Immunotherapy is not useful for eczema, food allergy, vasomotor rhinitis, and chronic hives. Allergy shots are most useful for hayfever and asthma.

584 **Bronchial Obstruction under 18 Months of Age**

Bronchial obstruction in children under 18 months of age is due mainly to mucosal edema and airway mucus, not bronchoconstrictions. Use daily inhaled steroids and cromolyn for prevention of inflammatory edema. Use albuterol for as-needed treatment for breakthroughs of other treatment.

585 **The Itch that Rashes**

Atopic dermatitis is not the rash that itches but the itch that rashes. Almost all severe cases of eczema are infected with staphylococci.

586 **Homicide in Black Males**

Homicide is the leading cause of death among black males aged 15–24 years.

587 **Youth Die Violent Deaths**

More youth, regardless of sex or race, die from violent means (suicide, accidents, and homicide) than from any other cause.

588 **Obesity and Antileukemia Therapy**

Obesity is both an early and late side effect of antileukemic therapy.

589 **Butchers Have Warts**

Butchers have more hand warts than people in any other profession. One wonders about their wives and children.

590 **Introduce People You Admire to Your Children**

Expose your children to people you admire. Let their enthusiasm rub off on the children.

591 **TSH Levels in Treatment of Hypothyroidism**

Early normalization of thyroid-stimulating hormone levels should be the goal in the treatment of hypothyroidism.

592 **Age of Baby and Onset of Congestive Heart Failure**

- < 7 days—aortic atresia
- 7–30 days—coarctation and patent ductus arteriosus
- 30–60 days—transposition

Contributed by Dr. John Phillips of Vanderbilt

593 **Date a Bruise**

Do you know how to date a bruise? If you have to testify in an abuse case, this table may be useful:

Criteria for Dating Bruises

Characteristics	Age of Bruise
Swollen, tender	0–2 days
Red, blue, purple	0–5 days
Green	5–7 days
Yellow	7–10 days
Brown	10–14 days
Clear	2–4 weeks

594 **Trusting Parents**

Lucky children enjoy the faith and trust of their parents. The best way to bring up children to do what is right is to show them that you know they will do what is right.

595 **Don't Punish Yourself Too**

Avoid statements such as, "If you don't take your medicine, we cannot go to the movie." This punishes everyone

596 **Our Friend, Fever**

- Fever is not our enemy but our friend.
- Fever is not a disease.
- Fever is beneficial and may be necessary for survival.
- Fever slows down the multiplication of bacteria and viruses.
- Fever increases the body's defense mechanism to fight infection.
- Tell parents that the height of the fever is not as important as what causes the fever.
- Reassure parents about fever!

597 **Pain that Wakes a Child**

Worry about all pain that awakens a child from sleep.

598 **Goiter: Think TSH Level**

If palpation raises the suspicion of goiter, thyroid-stimulating hormone level is usually the only test necessary.

599 **Backward Urination**

To get a midstream clean urine from an older girl, have her sit on the toilet backward to void. This position spreads the labia well.

600 **Pearls Outside the Hospital**

Dr. Osler said, "Medicine is learned by the bedside and not in the classroom." In pediatrics only 5% of practice is in the hospital. Most of the pearls in this book were learned outside the hospital.

INDEX

Note: Numbers refer to pearl number—there are no page numbers.